Personal Dispatches

Michael Denneny, General Editor

Stonewall Inn Editions

Buddies by Ethan Mordden
Joseph and the Old Man by Christopher Davis
Blackbird by Larry Duplechan
Gay Priest by Malcolm Boyd
Privates by Gene Horowitz
Taking Care of Mrs. Carroll by Paul Monette
Conversations with My Elders by Boze Hadleigh
Epidemic of Courage by Lon Nungesser
One Last Waltz by Ethan Mordden
Gay Spirit by Mark Thompson
As If After Sex by Joseph Torchia
The Mayor of Castro Street by Randy Shilts
Nocturnes for the King of Naples by Edmund White
Alienated Affections by Seymour Kleinberg
Sunday's Child by Edward Phillips
The God of Ecstasy by Arthur Evans
Valley of the Shadow by Christopher Davis
Love Alone by Paul Monette
The Boys and Their Baby by Larry Wolff
On Being Gay by Brian McNaught
Parisian Lives by Samuel M. Steward
Living the Spirit by Will Roscoe, ed.
Everybody Loves You by Ethan Mordden
Untold Decades by Robert Patrick
Gay and Lesbian Poetry in Our Time by Carl Morse and Joan Larkin, eds.
Reports from the holocaust: the making of an AIDS activist by Larry Kramer
Personal Dispatches by John Preston, ed.
Tangled Up in Blue by Larry Duplechan

Stonewall Inn Mysteries

Death Takes the Stage by Donald Ward
Sherlock Holmes and the Mysterious Friend of Oscar Wilde by Russell A. Brown
A Simple Suburban Murder by Mark Richard Zubro

Personal Dispatches

WRITERS CONFRONT AIDS

EDITED BY
John Preston

ST. MARTIN'S PRESS
NEW YORK

(Permissions continued on page 184)

Library of Congress Cataloging-in-Publication Data

Personal dispatches : writers confront AIDS / edited by John Preston.
    p.   cm.
    ISBN 0-312-05141-7 (pbk.)
    1. AIDS (Disease)—Literary collections.   2. American
literature—20th century.   3. Gay men—Literary collections.
4. Gays' writings, American.   I. Preston, John.
PS509.A43P4   1989
810.8'356—dc20   89-35320

FIRST PAPERBACK EDITION: November 1990

10 9 8 7 6 5 4 3 2 1

IN MEMORIUM

Stephen Chapot
November 21, 1951–August 24, 1988

Steven Franklin Marco ("Steve")
July 12, 1941–August 2, 1988

For some of us must storm
the castles
Some define the happening
—Arthur Nortje

Diane Elze of Maine ACT-UP; Gregory Gazaway of Boston ACT-OUT; Dale McCormick of the Maine Lesbian and Gay Political Alliance; Veneita Porter, Director of the Office on AIDS Discrimination for the State of New York; Eric Rofes, Executive Director of the Shanti Project of San Francisco; and Patrick Rumrill of ACT-UP of Washington State are some of the people I admire most for their relentless energy and clear-thinking action in response to the AIDS crisis.

I gratefully dedicate this book to them, to ACT-UP, and to the whole army of AIDS activists who have done so much to change the world in which we live.

—J.P.

CONTENTS

ACKNOWLEDGMENTS

The Introduction documents the many people who suggested articles for inclusion in this volume. I'm very indebted to them all for their help.

All the contributors to the book have been not only professional but also very kind and gentle in their dealings with me, which I appreciate very much.

Jonathan Ambrosino, Stephen Greco, Tom Hagerty, Robert Riger, and Bob Summer read drafts of my own essays and made effective comments that I valued.

My cousin Ann Hilferty was a great role model in my youth. She burst out of a childhood in working-class Somerville, Massachusetts, and into a brilliant international career as an educator. By her example, she showed a whole generation of our extended family what the possibilities of our lives could be. Anne and I lost track of one another for many years and have only recently remade contact. Part of getting to know one another again has been her intensive critique of the Introduction, which she so graciously gave me and which greatly improved my writing. Working as a colleague with her showed me that I, indeed, have become an adult, and it's added a special layer of self-awareness to the entire business of making this book.

Tom Hagerty also supplied endless hours of proofreading

and clerical labor as I worked to turn an idea into a manuscript and finally into a finished book. His belief in the importance of this collection was often the fuel I needed to continue. Tom has had this role of clerical and literary helpmate in many other projects of mine. It's always at the end of an undertaking that I fully understand just how important his assistance has been. His lover, André Roberge, has made his own offerings by allowing the outlandish demands I've often made on Tom's time and energy, and we both thank André for that.

My agent, Peter Ginsberg, and his assistant, Karen Nazor, have both made life as easy as possible for a demanding client. It is a great coincidence that Karen's father, Hugh Nazor, and her stepmother, Linda Murnik, are my landlords and friends. It's given the making of this book another dimension as a communal undertaking, and I think we've all done quite well using the advantages the situation offered, just as we've avoided the difficulties it could have presented.

Michael Denneny and I have been close comrades and collaborators for more than ten years. It's wonderfully satisfying that we finally have had a chance to work on a book together and that it is one so important to both of us. I've valued having him as an editor; it's shown me that he is just as good at his trade as he is at friendship.

Keith Kahla and Sarah Pettit, Michael's assistants at St. Martin's, have helped greatly by doing all those good works that editorial assistants can perform to make the publishing process as easy as possible.

All of these consultants, contributors, and readers have helped to make this a collaborative effort. Their good fellowship in the construction of this anthology displays the best of what a literary community might be. I thank everyone very much for making this an exciting experience.

—J. P.

INTRODUCTION

But, sure, the bravery of his grief did put me
Into a tow'ring passion

—Hamlet, V, ii

Two years ago, in 1986, a young bodybuilder came and asked whether he could pose for me. I had had some success as a physique photographer years ago when I lived in Manhattan, and a magazine he contacted had suggested he approach me to see if I would be interested in taking his picture.

I loved photographic work and regretted not pursuing it more strongly after I moved here, so I always accept these opportunities when they arise.

The session was successful. I was excited by the play of shadows the Maine winter light had created on his smooth skin. These photographs, I was sure, would be much more than the technically good snapshots that make up most male erotica. The model and I had worked well together. I knew there was something powerful in the session. I idly wondered if that ill-defined additional ingredient came from the physical attraction I felt for him, animated by this intimate encounter during which I'd been able to move his naked body about at my whim.

At the end, after he'd cleaned up and dressed, we sat at my dining room table and talked. He was about twenty-seven, a country boy from New Brunswick, Canada, who'd spent many hours in the gym building up a handsome body. He told me he had dreamed of a career as a model. I asked him if that was the reason he had decided to do the photographs for this magazine. I wasn't convinced that appearing naked in a glossy publication was the way to professional success.

"No, that's not it," he said suddenly. His eyes began to tear. "I just found out I have AIDS and I want them all to remember me when I was beautiful."

He broke down then. I gave him what comfort I could and listened as he told me his story. He'd just been diagnosed and he was concerned that his attractiveness, the one thing he'd always been able to count on, was going to go soon. There were warnings about KS lesions and almost a certainty of weight loss. He no longer had the energy for his strenuous workouts and his muscle tone would soon fade. His body had been his one great work of art and now he was going to lose it along with everything else. He wanted a totem of who he had become before the disease took over, and his photographs in a national magazine were the best answer he could come up with.

". . . I want them all to remember me when I was beautiful. . . ."

When he left, I sat in the apartment and cried and felt something happen to me. It was then, that evening when I was alone, that my heart broke, and I wasn't sure I could ever put it back together again.

It wasn't just him; it was what was happening to all of us. The string of this one story suddenly pulled together my grief for every one of the people I'd known over the years who had suffered because of AIDS.

By 1986, any gay man who had lived during the 1970s in New York or San Francisco or Los Angeles knew too many people with AIDS. And I had lived in all three cities during that decade. I had visited too many hospitals, had received too many late-night panicked phone calls, had read too many obituaries of too many friends. The idea of being able to cope with the AIDS epidemic was finally gone. This one episode became the focal point for my utter exhaustion and the erosion of my spirit.

As I sat alone that night, I wondered how I could possibly endure this. The poignancy of this young man's attempt to be remembered struck me powerfully.

It was a short while later that I picked up a copy of *Bay Windows* and read E. J. Graff's interview with the Politanos ("Bring Them Home"). My own life has left me with few illusions about the reactions of biological families; most of the families I knew of had acted horribly when confronted with their children's disease. I looked through the romantic appeal of the article, with its promise of limitless parental support, and saw instead its severe, unblinking look at the realities of AIDS, the descriptions of what it was like to feed someone and clean him and listen to him while he was dying.

There was something empowering in reading that piece, in seeing that description and understanding that people could, indeed, persist in providing that witness. This seemed to me a new form of AIDS writing. It wasn't about the politics of the disease; it wasn't about the twisted machinations of the Centers for Disease Control or the National Institutes of Health; it wasn't self-pitying or alarmist; and it certainly wasn't escapist. It was writing which acknowledged the extreme realities of AIDS. It looked the calamity in the face; it told how people had survived the illness and death of a loved one; and it was honest.

I wanted to read more writing about AIDS that had this integrity. I made a few inquiries and asked people what they had seen that had touched this raw nerve. Jim Baxter, the editor of *The Front Page* in North Carolina, sent me two articles by Allan Troxler ("Wandering the Woods in a Season of Death" and "A Letter Home on Pride Day"). Here again was a writer grappling with the most personal issues of the epidemic. Here was a man who responded to a friend's illness and struggled with the pain it brought, only to find out, a year later, that the illness had moved even closer, to claim the life of his lover.

Mark Thompson, an editor of *The Advocate*, sent back an envelope with Arnie Kantrowitz's "Friends Gone with the Wind," noting that it had generated more response mail than any other one piece in the magazine's history. It had touched readers' lives through its passionate report of how this one writer in New York was coping with the disease as it stormed around him. First-person testimonies like the Politanos' are vital, but the reflections of writers like Kantrowitz upon the effect of the plague on politics and other aspects of modern life provoke a thoughtfulness I wanted to encourage, in myself and in others. To grieve for a person—to grieve for my aspiring model or for John Politano—is a real response to AIDS. But it is important to understand the context within which these personal events are occurring. This certainly is one of the most important roles of a writer in the midst of a maelstrom as devastating as this medical crisis, and people like Kantrowitz were providing it.

Mark Thompson also sent me a copy of Robert Glück's "HTLV-3," an article about the dilemma so many people were facing, including myself: Should we be tested? Were we better off knowing whether or not we were infected with the incurable virus, or should we just go on living with our unspeakable anxiety and worry? (HTLV-3 would later be renamed HIV by an international congress.) It is an elegant essay which speaks to an issue which still concerns many people years later. The insights Glück gives to the decision and the fear it represents are powerful.

The same package from Mark Thompson contained a third piece, Edmund White's "Esthetics and Loss." I especially had looked forward to reading White's assessment of how we writers should proceed in response to AIDS. The virus gives no respite; it makes you pay emotionally for the chances to have this kind of contemplation; it doesn't accommodate investigation with academic distance. I saw that as soon as I began to read about the young artist whom White portrays. How could I have been prepared to read about the death of Kris Johnson, one of my first loves?

I was shaken by the news, not just because it was such an extreme loss, but because it showed me still another way in which I was being deprived by the pestilence. My relationship with Kris, nearly twenty years earlier, had never seemed to resolve itself. I had always kept track of him somewhat; while I hadn't known he was sick, I knew that he'd moved to New Mexico.

I had a fantasy about Kris, one that a man my age should have been able to hold: that we would meet sometime and at least talk about what had happened between us. Perhaps we could even start again, so my dream went, but at least we could talk about what had happened. Now he was gone, and it wasn't just that *he* was gone, but that all these men I had loved were dead and their connection with me was left hanging in the air, their spirits unresolved, the possibilities left unrealized.

I became overwhelmed by the numbers of people who were lost—from my own life, from the gay community, from the art world, from all of our lives. As I read these articles, I was able finally to begin to grasp the size of the tragedy of AIDS. Its scope awed me. Its scale staggered me. I don't believe I ever really denied that any of this was happening—as a journalist I certainly knew the statistics—but this new reading focused all these issues for me in a way that was far more powerful than the recitation of data.

It was at that point that I decided in earnest to make a book of these articles. I had constructed anthologies before; here was the base for a new one. I would ask other authors to contribute essays. Along with these I'd already collected, I could make a book that could register the beauty and the strength of these people who were living with AIDS, either with the disease itself or with its effects on them and the world around them.

I wrote to more than a dozen people I had worked with on other projects and asked for contributions. At first, almost all said yes. Then I learned about a new shape of the illness: the paralysis that it can bring. Most of the deadlines passed unmet. I queried the writers involved and asked what problems they were having. Many simply never answered, which was uncharacteristic of them. Some of those who did reply confessed that they, or their lover, or their best friend had been diagnosed and they were incapable of writing about AIDS, at least for now. Even more admitted that they were so immobilized by the fear of AIDS that they simply couldn't write about it.

The disease was eating us up, taking away our energy, diverting writers from writing and forcing us to deal with daily emergencies that allowed few of us to create easily or meditate, making what was written all the more valuable.

One original piece did come out of those first queries. Steve Beery's "Steve" recognizes and validates the sexual and emotional lives of people who are living with AIDS. More, it documents how many of this epidemic's caregivers are themselves infected. Being the "buddy" of a person living with AIDS while he coped with the news of his own infection is a story I knew was being repeated over and over again.

I continued to ask people for suggestions for this book. I was struck, especially, by how much very good material was in small gay presses like *The Front Page*. I felt strongly that it should be set before a national audience.

When I explained that to Richard Labonté, who was then manager of A Different Light, the lesbian and gay bookstore in Los Angeles, he immediately suggested Stephen Chapot's "Liz Taylor, Live!"—a brilliant and angry depiction of a person with AIDS living through a Hollywood fundraiser. The piece had been published in San Diego's *UpDate*, one of the many gay newspapers that had begun as "bar rags"—little more than social calendars for the local taverns—but that had grown over the course of the years and out of the needs of the epidemic to become mature journals of information and opinion.

My friends told me that there was also writing going on which wasn't even being published but which was being handed around, friend to friend, as people found their own responses to AIDS and its symbols and tried to share them.

The March on Washington in October of 1987 brought The NAMES Project to national attention. The communal struggle with memory that it represented has produced the Quilt, the most powerful emblem to come from the AIDS epidemic. Michael Denneny sent me a copy of Robert Dawidoff's essay, a commentary which combines an academic deliberation on the meaning of the Quilt with a strong personal statement.

Dawidoff's expressions about the Quilt hit home because I had wandered up and down its pathways in Washington myself. I began to recognize the contributors to this book as fellow travelers, others who were on the front lines of the struggle with AIDS. I saw this book as something that I could present to others who wanted to see what were the real experiences coming from this horrible chapter in our lives. This is the truth, I could say to any reader, this is no melodramatic document. This is what we have been going through. I know. I was there with these writers.

I found another example in Laurence Tate's "The Epidemic: A San Francisco Diary" in *Arrival* magazine. I'd worked with many people in my home state to establish the Maine Health Foundation to provide money for AIDS services in our corner of the country. I'd worked with many people who provided direct services to people who were living with AIDS, and with the fear of it. I could see at once the precision and accuracy of Tate's discussion of what it means to work on an AIDS hotline. The stories of the volunteers who work to help people— through direct care, with information, whatever—deserve to be told and retold whenever the plague is mentioned.

The tightening circle of AIDS finally came too closely into my own life. In 1987, I received my own positive test for HIV antibodies; I learned that I was infected with the disease myself.

It was then that I truly understood the difficulties that many other writers had with their stories, and I became all the more admiring of those who would tell their truths. Because I couldn't do it, not for well over a year. The manuscript sat on a shelf in my study, something too raw for me to read, too difficult. The epidemic became more immediate, became suffocating, became the way I learned of my lovers' and friends' deaths. Now the book seemed, in its own strange way, to have become the harbinger of my own infection. Faced with pressing medical decisions and a sense of dread about the repercussions of having AIDS in today's society, it seemed there was no time to create a book, there was no relief from the oppression of the illness. How could one reflect on all that was happening *when it was happening now*?

But, in fact, this collection was one of the means I had at my disposal to come back to life. These articles had helped me fight the feeling that AIDS was overwhelming me. The writers with whom I was working were dealing with the disease, each in his or her own way, as the infected or the care providers, as the givers of testimony or as the interpreters of history. It seemed an ever more appropriate community for me. I could see, even more clearly now, how all the writers in this book were participant/observers in the plague. The power of their pieces came from their ability not to withdraw from the disaster but to encounter it, to send dispatches back from their personal trenches and to give their messages to the world. My response couldn't be to withdraw into my own personal fears. That would mean turning myself into a victim who had no will, no affect on what was happening around and to him. It would mean the passive acceptance of the infection as the end of my life. As a writer, I could at least reassert myself as one of the participant/observers. I could be part of recording what this epidemic was doing to my world, only now in a different role than the one I'd first envisioned for myself.

I met with Michael Bronski, a mainstay of Boston's *Gay Community News (GCN)*, and received tremendous support in my resolve to continue with the project. Bronski also gave me two of his published articles, which helped me to define once again the importance of this writing I was pulling together. Bronski's "AIDS, Art and Obits" was exactly the kind of writing for which I was looking. What does it mean to type out the endless eulogies for the fallen? What does it do to a writer?

Bronski's "Death and the Erotic Imagination" had been originally printed in *Radical America*. It dared to investigate forbidden subjects and their interconnectedness in a way, that illuminated my own understanding and my own life.

In *Drummer* magazine, I found an early version of Scott Tucker's "Well, Was It Worth It?"—another essay that dealt directly with how AIDS was not just consuming us with sorrow but also was being used to attack our sexuality.

I discovered that Andrew Holleran had an essay on "The Fear," which hadn't yet been published. When I read the manuscript, I realized that the piece was addressing many of the elements that were clearly becoming so important to me, especially the lucidity of many people who were infected as opposed to some of those who were the "worried well," a distinction I now could comprehend much more clearly.

Stephen Greco is someone I knew professionally—we had worked together while he had been an editor at *The Advocate*— but he was also a friend. I remember we had shared lunch once after his lover, Barry Laine, died. Stephen had asked me if I had ever gotten over the death of my own lover, Jason Klein, who'd died—not of AIDS—years earlier. He wanted to know what it would be like to live with his own mourning over Barry's death. We'd discussed the value of our grief. We talked about how we didn't want to have it "healed" or to have it "go away" or to stop, because it was too significant to be denied. But one had to go on, I explained to Stephen, and the way I'd learned how was to encapsulate the grief, to put it in a special place in my memory so I could bring it down and open it up when it was important to remember and to feel those emotions again.

A long time after that discussion, I read his "Excerpts from a

Journal," which had appeared in the *European Gay Review*. I knew it was vital to have this record of a lover's experience as part of this book. The deaths of lovers and spouses have been the stuff of literature throughout history, of course. But AIDS is forcing so many of us to deal with this loss at such an early age. Greco and his lover were in the prime of their lives when the illness swept Barry up. The obituaries of the people we love come as hard and often to those of us who are touched by AIDS as they do to our grandparents.

There are some who object to the analogy of the struggle against AIDS to war. They feel it's inappropriate to connect a medical happening with a military campaign. But there is one way in which the analogy is all too appropriate. AIDS is like war in the way it insults nature. It reverses the order of life and death: the elders burying the younger generation. We who survive live with the announcements of the deaths of people who are too often younger than we are. It's certainly true for me. Of the dozens of people dead of AIDS whom I knew well, all of them—all of those beautiful men whose photographs inundate my memory—were younger than I when they died.

This book also had to contain something about the experience of people living with AIDS and the medical system. I knew that the way people are caught up in the establishment once they are diagnosed is one of the most intense topics among people who have HIV infections. Craig Rowland had earned insights into all of that and I encouraged him to write them up in "The Examination Table."

Marea Murray has long been a hero of AIDS work in Boston and her chronicling of the disease and how people react to it in *GCN* has constituted some of the best AIDS writing in that important publication. Her article displays the great contributions that lesbians have given to the struggles against the illness in all its forms. Murray's chronicle of her work also provides a chance to point to one of the truisms about AIDS in our society: While gay men have, so far, been those who have been most able to give witness to what has gone on, this disease is also striking hard at people of color, at women and their children. AIDS knows no ghettos, it has no sexual preference, and it has no morality.

As I come to the end of the work of assembling this anthology, Murray's exhaustion rings true, tells me and the world what I feel most about this whole enterprise. Her determined looking forward, finding the same hope in people's courage that Arnie Kantrowitz insisted upon in the first essay in this collection, is our only possible option, weary or not.

Finally, Robert Dawidoff wrote another original piece for this anthology, a memorandum of a dialogue with Michael Denneny, which actually serves as the apologia for this book. The goals that he describes and the imperatives he outlines are the reasons why I think this volume should exist.

These are voices of people who are in the midst of the AIDS epidemic, the caregivers, the people living with AIDS, the infected, the activists, the interpreters. These are the images I and my collaborators have created of our own and other people's lives during the time of AIDS. There is anger here, and immeasurable grief. There is celebration and hope and there is witness to those who have been here and what they have gone through. There is truth in this book, as we, the writers, have experienced it. I hope that truth will empower other readers as much as it has me.

JOHN PRESTON
Portland, Maine
November 1988

A note to the reader: Some of these essays were published as early as 1985. The facts and figures of AIDS have changed dramatically in those few years. This book is not intended as a primer on AIDS. There's been no attempt to "update" the information with which the authors worked. A bibliography of books about AIDS and the phone numbers of AIDS organizations that can give you current information are included in *You Can Do Something About AIDS*, a volume underwritten by the publishing industry and available free from most bookstores.

As of March 1, 1990, 128,319 people in the United States had been diagnosed with AIDS; 78,341 of them had died. The Surgeon General has estimated that one and a half million Americans have been infected with HIV, the virus he believes causes AIDS; research suggests that most of those will develop AIDS. No one knows for sure.

Personal Dispatches

Prologue

These are three days of being a writer in the midst of the AIDS epidemic. . . .

I woke up on Wednesday excited after returning from a trip to New York; I'd just gotten back to Maine late the night before. I'd met with Michael Denneny at St. Martin's Press while I'd been in the city and he had expressed real enthusiasm for the first draft of the manuscript of this anthology. There's a tremendous excitement in the creation of a book, and it'd taken me more than two years to accomplish this one.

But something was very wrong and I couldn't really get going that morning. I was woozy, wrung out, and a long night's sleep hadn't refreshed me. I'd felt rotten the whole four days I'd been in Manhattan, but I put that down to the pace of the city. I moved to Maine eight years ago, and I wasn't used to the fast-lane excitement anymore, I tried to convince myself. Or was it the beginning of middle age? I'm forty-two, old enough not to be running around as much as I used to. Had I had too much to drink during all the Halloween celebrations and rich dinners? No. Everything's done in moderation now, so that didn't make any sense.

But I did feel awful.

I began the business of contacting the contributors, calling some with the good news from St. Martin's and telling them that I'd be printing out my typescripts of their articles for their proofreading; writing to some others who hadn't yet gotten me their final drafts, to urge them to hurry up; giving out new deadlines; doing all that kind of business.

I welcomed all the activity, but I kept an eye on the clock,

1

waiting until I could call Massachusetts General Hospital in Boston. Nine months ago, I'd volunteered for an experimental study they were doing to see if something couldn't stop the disease from progressing in people like myself who are HIV-positive—asymptomatic carriers of the virus that causes AIDS. The results of my most recent blood tests were to be in late in the day and I wanted to get ahold of them.

When I finally got through that afternoon, Graham, the nurse who administers the program, answered. It's very seldom that medicine comes up with an elegant word, but I already knew I was suffering rrom what the doctors call *malaise*. Such a descriptive term. I recited the symptoms to her. "It's not surprising, your 'crit is awfully low."

We all speak in jargon nowadays, and I knew she meant the measurements for my red-blood count must be far below normal. Did that mean anything about my T_4 cells, the indicators of the deterioration of one's immune system?

She read off my numbers. I'd been through this dozens of times and I knew how to translate the figures. The T_4s were okay—far fewer than a half of what a really healthy person would have, but the drop from the last test wasn't very dramatic. We could ascribe it to the regular fluctuations in the measurement. T_4 counts can be maddeningly volatile; it's such a vital calculation of one's health, but it can often move up and down the scale with no apparent meaning.

The rest of the results weren't so good. I was anemic; that's why I had been feeling so awful; my body was rejecting AZT, the drug I was taking. The drug sometimes poisons your bone marrow, cutting off the production of red-blood cells, among other things. It had already happened once before during the summer. I was a pro at this now. I knew I had to get a new blood test done right away to see whether there had been any more change in my red-cell count. I might need a transfusion to heal myself. This second bout with AZT toxicity also meant that my continued participation in the study was questionable.

Did I even want to continue, though? That was a more pressing question.

I talked to a specialist, who termed the decision "major league." It certainly was that. There is nothing else I could take at this point. Of course, I could work with my nutrition and wonder about alternative therapies, but AZT is the only thing in the traditional medical arsenal that doctors feel comfortable prescribing. AZT has been shown to add significant time to the lives of people with terminal AIDS symptoms. The whole purpose of this program for which I'd volunteered was to determine whether the drug would help those of us who are infected but not yet showing symptoms, or whether the toxicity was so great that the drug wasn't worth our taking it.

After I hung up, I felt my body begin to fail. I realized what was going on right away. I don't want to be sick. I still try to ignore the messages of weakness my body sends to me. That's what had been happening to me in New York, I understood. I had refused to give in to the fatigue and the anemia the drug had been producing; I wanted to make believe everything was all right. I didn't want to admit to experiencing anything that had something to do with AIDS or with its drugs.

But once I had heard the numbers, then my defenses began to fall. The evidence was in front of me. Yes, I was sick. It wasn't AIDS, but it was real. I let the waves of exhaustion and sadness roll over me and I collapsed into bed, wanting to stay there for a week.

The phone rang. I sat up, suddenly alert, as a voice told me a friend had been admitted to Osteopathic Hospital here in Portland while I was gone. I called Joe at once.

"Where have you *been?!*" Joe was angry with me for being away when he'd gotten sick. He is one of the most difficult clients at The AIDS Project, his rough manner turns off many other people at the same time it endears him to me. He's full of

3

fear and hurt after a horde of cancers and infections and other diseases have invaded and attacked his body. I might be obsessive about my own falling T_4 cell count, but my numbers are in the hundreds and to recite them to Joe when his own count was 84—the last time they bothered to check—makes me into a braggart. I talked as calmly as I could and coaxed him into telling me what was wrong. He had an intestinal virus. He had been barely able to eat or move his bowels since he'd been admitted on Saturday.

The story was all delivered with a sharp edge to it. Joe is defiant, furious with the idea that he might die soon. What can I possibly do about it?

"Is there anything you want?"

"I can't eat anything." Joe whines after he has your attention. He's twenty-five now, but when this happens, he turns into a bratty little boy; there's something sniffling about his manner.

"You have to eat, you know that."

"I can't hold anything down. They put it in, I throw it up."

"Joe, is there anything I can bring you that you'll eat?"

There was a silence. "Tootsie Rolls." I wanted to yell at him: *Don't pull this shit on me now, Joe. I can't take it. I'm exhausted. . . .* I was astonished by the surge of exasperation I felt toward him. *Why now, Joe? Why today?* I stopped myself. Joe never chose any of this; he certainly didn't decide the timing.

"Do you think you could eat them if I go to a store and get some for you?"

"I love Tootsie Rolls," he answered.

Joe has no other way to ask for anything of importance. He can only deal with these most primitive symbols. Asking me to bring him Tootsie Rolls is asking me to love him, and I do love him, so I drove to the market and got a jumbo bag.

While some people complain about Joe, I understand all of this. I've done the same things myself. I remember once, just after I'd received my own diagnosis, I had *demanded* that my friend Anne buy me a copy of *Dirty Dancing*. The videotape was just being released and it was going to be available in her home in San Francisco before it would reach Maine. I *had* to have a copy, I told her. She *had* to go out and buy one and Federal Express it to me. There was no choice in the matter. She was dazed by the force of the requirement, but she must have understood that asking for that videotape was all I could do at that moment. In the midst of my need and fear, those were the only words I could find. I wanted more from her; I wanted to ask the same things Joe was asking me now: *Help me. Love me. Tell me this is going to be all right.* But we can't articulate those pleas all the time, and so we ask for videotapes and we buy Tootsie Rolls—and we hope it helps everyone concerned.

Another friend was visiting when I finally got to Joe's hospital room. I sat down and listened to Michael's wonderful stories about "Miss Joe" and his past, his youth as a lobsterman Down East on the coast of Maine, his foolish encounters with men, his broken hearts and healed spirits. Michael's sharp queeny wit entertained us and brought me up out of my depression. I reveled in the good cheer he shared with both Joe and me. I was happy I had gone out there and had the time with both of them.

I drove home, at last, and fell to sleep.

Thursday, the next morning, I went to the walk-in clinic where Dale works. Dale and I had an eerily intimate relationship. She'd drawn the blood that had produced my diagnosis. Before I'd entered the study at Mass General, she'd been the one who'd taken the blood for my regular T_4 counts.

The clinic staff knows that Dale will always be the one to see me. We're established as a pair. I've no doubts that the other nurses would do anything necessary—there's no hint in this urban clinic that they would turn away anyone with an HIV infection—but Dale and I are assumed. As soon as I walk in the doors, they tell me her schedule and rearrange whatever must be done to get me to see her as efficiently as possible.

I already knew I looked bad. The mirror showed the pallor of my skin. Dale only glanced at how pale I was and knew something was wrong.

I went into the examination room and sprawled on the couch, automatically lifting up my sleeve and baring my skin. Dale knows how much I hate the needle and we've long ago set up the procedure that I lie down for the test. We talked about my health and my fears about the infection. I'm scared now that the drug is just too much for me. I've given it nine months; it's done no demonstrable good; I don't want to go on feeling this way.

Dale swabbed the inside of my elbow with alcohol to clean it. She always tries to be upbeat and positive, but there was real concern in her voice as she questioned me about the specialists' opinions.

Finally, as I looked away—I hate the sight of my blood being taken from my body—the needle pricked. It was the first time Dale had ever missed my veins. "Oh, John, I'm sorry!" She sounded more surprised and hurt than I was and spoke with the passion of a lover who made a wrong move and was startled that it could ever have happened. She had to start again, probing painfully to find the usually cooperative vein.

It was done and the sample would be sent to the lab. I sat on the couch and we kept on talking, mainly about fear but also about the strangeness of having been made so sick for so long by something that was supposed to save my life. The melodrama of my words seemed to hurt her and she suddenly grabbed hold of me, embracing me warmly, even more caringly than she'd been doing all through these many months.

That night I continued talking to people involved with this book. One of the calls I made was to Scott Tucker.

Scott was worried about his article appearing as it originally had been published, without any reference to his own health status; he's also HIV-positive.

I remember when Scott and I first talked to one another about our positive test results, how thrown we were, wondering what to do, how to handle it. We'd each had a hard time of it because so many people *expected* us to have AIDS. We both published in sex magazines as well as "correct" literary journals. I'd written erotic books; he'd taken a fling and entered and won a national male beauty contest. We were two sexual outlaws of the Seventies, the ones who were supposed to get sick, so we were told, so people acted toward us. Now we were both infected and had to fend off the judgments that we "deserved" this illness.

Over the past eighteen months, I had slowly begun to tell other people about my infection. Many of them were friends like Scott, who I learned were also infected. We became a special kind of telephone link with one another: Scott in Philadelphia, another friend in Los Angeles, Steve Beery in San Francisco, Patrick in Tacoma, each one having whispered conversations during the night with me, talking about fear, not just of being ill and possibly dying but of both the political and the personal backlash of other people finding out about our status. It was an intimate web we created, a place where we could try out ideas we didn't always trust others to understand and where feelings were expressed that we didn't expect others to comprehend.

Scott and I both have been activists for years. Holding in a secret about ourselves went against the grain of two partisans who had learned that the personal was political. We wondered how to "come out" about our infections and told each other of our moves and our actions when we checked in for these special conversations.

I told him that night about my own decision to write this essay, and he was greatly relieved. His article and the integrity of his feelings and self-awareness when he wrote it could stand more easily if I was going to write about our health in this section.

Then Scott told me that he had decided to enter the same drug test I was just leaving. A teaching hospital in Philadelphia was replicating the research Mass General was undertaking.

All of my own turmoil rose to the surface. We discussed the possibilities of the drug. I understood his desire for an active intervention. I'd had the same craving myself when I had entered the Mass General study.

But it was going to be difficult, I told him. There was no need to think that he was condemned to the toxic reactions I'd experienced; few of the participants had such an intense response. It was true, as well, that he would gain access to some of the top research specialists in the disease—one of my own motivations for entering the study. I couldn't hold any of that against him, even as I felt a jealousy building in anticipation of his doing well with the drug I had such a hard time accepting into my body.

Why take an experimental drug under these circumstances? We both knew the answer to that. It was a question of trying to add years to your life. He had been reading as much as he could about HIV and we both knew the risks of AZT; but the outlook is so bleak—the projected percentages of people who are infected with HIV who are predicted to die of AIDS seem to climb all the time, and some action seemed necessary.

We talked about what it was like to go into these medical centers. It wasn't an easy visit to a physician's office. It was much different. Crossing the threshold into a huge institution like Mass General brings an enormous sense of being swept up in the medical establishment, of being lost in it. The individual researchers try hard to be kind, but the pressures of the numbers of people waiting to get in to see them are simply too great. They try to give you time and to answer your questions, I explained to Scott, but they can't do it, not well enough for people like him and me, people who have challenges and who want complex responses.

8

I also told him one of the great dangers that I was only just then understanding. AZT is out there and people who are infected with HIV count on it—I had, he was. We all knew it would be there if it was needed, or when it was needed. There are great scientific debates going on about its use, whether or not its toxicity is so great that in the long run it might not be a good idea at all. But it's *there*. It may be tarnished, but it's still a magic bullet of sorts. I had never been warned that one of the results of my being in the test would be to discover that I shouldn't take the drug. That was what the evidence was showing me, that it was too dangerous for me now, and might be in the future.

It seemed so poignant, that conversation with Scott, one friend beginning a path with hope while another one left the same track and felt vulnerable, unprotected against the virus.

It was too much. My fatigue hadn't abated at all. After more than an hour, I hung up and slept.

Friday morning, Dale called and gently told me that my blood counts from the test the day before were significantly lower than when they'd been taken at Mass General. I called Boston and talked to Graham. I could either have a transfusion and see about taking up the drug again later or I could drop out of the study. It wasn't an irrational choice to leave the drug behind, she agreed, not with this toxicity.

We made arrangements for me to continue to be monitored by the specialists at Mass General. After the past nine months, I was of value to them. They would want to see what my body did once it no longer was receiving AZT. I could talk to the head researcher on one of my next visits to Boston. He'd explore my other options with me then.

There aren't very many. I wondered about getting dextran sulfate from Japan. Washington won't let it be sold in this country but it will allow infected people to import it—an example of "compassion" in the federal policy. I couldn't possibly afford it myself. Insurance won't pay for such a quasilegal drug. There are rumors coming eastward from California, where it's gained some popularity, of its cwn toxicity. I didn't want to think about it more—I had to meet Pam, my GP, at the lawyer's office.

I had to put aside my work on this book. I had another kind of writing to do.

It was just happenstance that I had set up this appointment to have my will drawn and other legal documents signed on this day. I should have done it long ago, and even after I had acted, it had taken a while to get everything written up and for schedules to be coordinated.

Laurel, the attorney to whom The AIDS Project had sent me, explained that in Maine a person with a life-threatening disease should have a physician witness the signing of documents like a will. Otherwise, they were too open to challenge; the diagnosis could be seen as a kind of de facto duress if a doctor hadn't been there to certify the person's competence. It wasn't just a will that was involved. I also needed a medical power of attorney so my friends can make decisions if I ever get sick, and there were other legal papers that were necessary for them to act on my behalf in case I were incapacitated. Pam had agreed to come into the city to do the witnessing.

I met her at Laurel's office. Pam was carrying her new son, Benjamin. I'd never seen him before. He was three months old, smiling, a happy baby. Pam spread out his blanket and put him on the floor to play while the adult business went on.

It was remarkably complicated, no matter how easy Laurel tried to make it. Certain papers had to be notarized; still another witness had to be present when Pam and I signed some of the affidavits. There was traffic in and out of the office as the appropriate people came and went.

Laurel and Pam kept the conversation focused on the future.

Laurel talked about what would happen to those documents she was to keep in case she was to move in two years; Pam talked about the changes in the law and treatment five years ahead.

Why shouldn't we talk that way? An HIV infection can linger in this dormant stage for a decade, perhaps longer. Some people—no one knows how many—may live a full lifetime. In any event, Pam has always insisted that as her patient, I aspire to beat all the odds. No matter how much we tried, however, I couldn't escape the sensation that we were preparing for my death with all of these papers. Then there was this strange moment when Laurel had to ask Pam out loud whether she deemed me competent to make these decisions. Suddenly it all seemed surreal—to have my capability to control my life so boldly questioned.

I looked at Benjamin lying on the floor. He was so small, but his adult features were coming through, and I could see him growing up, a cocky kid, living in a context of obvious adoration from his mother and, I was sure, his father, another physician.

At some moment while all the legal transactions were going on, Pam suddenly said, "Look, he's holding his bottle with both hands! That's something new. A small moment in history."

Benjamin had the bottle clutched in his fists. He seemed to be staring back at me, his eyes full of laughter. He threw his hands up in the air and let the bottle go, but only smiled more broadly, holding his arms up in the air, as though he were a gymnast who'd just performed the perfect dismount, ready to accept the cheers of the crowd.

Then it was over.

Pam and Benjamin and I took the elevator down to the lobby of the building. We stood there and talked about the decision to go off the drug. I had begun it with the same hope Scott held, that it would prolong my life. Now, after the past nine months, a period during which I'd never felt really well, I wanted out.

Pam stood there and held Benjamin in her arms while I explained how I felt, even with my lowering T_4 cells. As always, she was clear and concise. "Everyone with a chronic disease like an HIV infection has to make choices between quantity and quality all the time. That's what you're doing. No one knows that the AZT would have worked, and no one can tell you that you're going to do worse without it. Remember, your blood is part of your immune system as well. It's been impaired by this drug. Who knows, perhaps it's just as important that you let your body heal and let it do its own work.

"The big thing is for you to choose the best quality of life. That's what you've done and I can support that in every way." Benjamin smiled his agreement, his small fists reaching out of his blanket and punching the air with innocent enthusiasm. We all said good night to one another.

Then we parted and I came home and went to sleep, thinking about how I was going to complete this book. . . .

Friends Gone with the Wind

ARNIE KANTROWITZ

I am in a strange apartment in the Bronx, stretched out on a double *chaise longue*, waiting for Hitler's funeral to begin. My dear friend Malcolm (I'm changing some names for privacy's sake) appears in the doorway and makes his way toward me through the crowd. He lies down next to me, but when I turn to kiss him hello, I discover that he has been transformed into a withered old woman. She smiles. The funeral begins.

With tears in my eyes, I wake up. The horror of AIDS has finally penetrated my unconscious, and I know that now there is no escape from reality, not even in sleep.

Fantasy has always been an escape valve for me. When I was at my lowest ebb or when I just needed a rest from it all, I could always go to the movies. If I was especially lucky, *Gone With the Wind* would be showing somewhere in town, and I could struggle along with Scarlett O'Hara through love and loss and sweeping change and, mustering my fortitude and determination, declare along with her, "As God is my witness, I'll never go hungry again," while stuffing buttered popcorn in my mouth.

In the urban gay ghetto of the 1970s, I found an even better escape. If an evening threatened to be empty or unpleasant, I could retreat to the phantasmagoria of the baths and back-room bars, wandering through an endless maze of rooms and corridors to act out my erotic dreams with partner after part-ner, imagining that the likes of Rhett Butler was waiting be-hind each zipper or under each towel. What a fabulous party it was! All the pent-up yearnings of our repressed youths were abandoned along with our clothes. We were inexhaustibly cre-ative and more sophisticated than everyone else, or so we fan-cied, unaware of our perilous innocence. We explored our dreams and our bodies as if we had invented sex for the very first time, helping countless unnamed men to orgasm, priv-ileged to live in the generation when freedom had at last ar-rived. We had no idea how swiftly history can repossess its gifts, how suddenly the enemy attacks.

At first it was a muffled rumble, like cannon fire in the dis-tance. My lover, Lawrence Mass, M.D., was the first person to write about AIDS outside of the medical press. He warned me that something monumental was about to happen, but it took a while for me to realize what he meant. I had heard that an *Advocate* editor, Brent, with whom I'd once had dinner in San Francisco, was dead.

Then others died. Ted, the owner of a well-known bar, whose former lover I'd had sex with several times. Billy—who'd delighted us all by dressing as a middle-aged matron at a garden party and singing old songs—was suddenly gone overnight, before anyone even knew he was ill. Eddie, the friend of a friend's friend. Howard, who'd produced gay con-sciousness-raising theater. Jack, whom I'd met at an esoteric orgy and who published an underground porn magazine. Pat-rick, the psychologist. Joe, the teacher. Lynne, the female im-personator. And Eric, whom I myself had had sex with, and Arthur, the lover of a friend, and Richard, the artist, and Peter, the political activist. There are eighteen gone as of this writing, and twelve others diagnosed, and four with AIDS-Related Complex (ARC).

(*Scarlett and Melanie are in the crowd at the newspaper office waiting for the lists of the dead and wounded at Gettysburg. Uncle Peter brings them one, torn by the crowd in its urgency.*)

RHETT: I'm sorry, Scarlett. (*She looks up at him.*) Many of your friends?

SCARLETT (*her voice choking*): "Just about every family in the country." (*She points to the list.*) " 'Calvert, Raiford, Lieutenant.' Raif! I grew up with Raif! 'Monroe, Joseph.' Little, bad-tempered Joe! And both of the Tarleton boys! Both of them, Rhett!" (*Even Scarlett breaks.*)

RHETT: "There'll be longer lists tomorrow and again the day after. And maybe for weeks to come."

SCARLETT (*miserably*): "Oh, Rhett, why do wars have to be?"

But fantasy can't keep the horror at its distance, of course. The circles grow even narrower, until I feel them at my very threshold.

Hank arrives at our door in tears. I hold him close. He has seen a close friend die, and now he has found a purple spot on his own side. Hank is lucky. The spot turns out to be nothing. But the fear is not nothing. It is great enough to send him into therapy.

Malcolm was not so lucky. First AIDS struck his former lover Frank, a childlike star-watcher who could name every Academy Award winner, year by year. Malcolm flew thousands of miles to be with him, living a real-life version of the story in William Hoffman's play *As Is*. Then Malcolm discovered a spot on his own leg, and the doctor had it biopsied. Another friend and I flew out to be with him. At first, the news came back good—only a mole—and we spent the weekend in the country, sighing with relief. But then more news came. The slides had been confused with those of an old woman from the Bronx. The spot was indeed Kaposi's sarcoma (KS). Malcolm's life turned upside down, and I began having nightmares.

(As Scarlett enters the railroad yard, all the horror and misery of what we are about to see are reflected in her face. The camera, drawing farther and farther back and upward, reveals the vast expanse of the depot—completely covered with the bodies of wounded soldiers. Only a handful of male orderlies and women attendants move amongst the wounded, some of whom lie stiff and still—others writhing under the hot sun. Involuntarily, her hand rises to her mouth as she fights back the quick nausea that hits her. Then, fighting her own desire to flee, to get away from this appalling scene, she forces herself to start through the rows of wounded. Everywhere the men are crying for water in a steady, low moan of voices.)

Most of us don't face the worst of life because we want to. We do it because we have to. So many of our people have proved to be heroic throughout this tribulation. In New York alone, there is a waiting list to join the 1,100 volunteers who visit people with AIDS—to offer comfort, shop for food, wash their floors, clean their vomit, and hold them while they cry. Some of these patients will face the worst of human experience before they die, losing sight and hearing and control of their bowels, forgetting their own names and suffering untold pain. But no matter how gruesome it gets, their brothers and sisters—from GMHC (Gay Men's Health Crisis) and San Francisco AIDS Foundation and AIDS Project Los Angeles and similar groups in San Diego, Seattle, Boston, and Miami, and elsewhere—are willing to stay beside them.

These are not stereotypical, flighty, sex-addicted faggots. These are humanity at its finest. Do our critics know how often we are society's servants, its comforters and nurturers? While they excoriate us for being frivolous fun-seekers, we work as nurses and therapists and teachers, beyond our proportions in the populace. There is more to the gay lifestyle than Sunday brunch. It takes nobility and perseverance and dignity and courage to be gay and proud in the face of condemnation and injustice, violence and death. I have never been so proud of our people as I am today.

I stopped partying as soon as I realized that my survival was at stake, and I settled down in a relationship. I gave money to Gay Men's Health Crisis. I talked about the epidemic in my writing. I went to benefits and rallies and candlelight marches.

But I didn't become a buddy and look after the sick. I didn't look the horror in the eye, so the horror came to me.

It burst upon the nation with Rock Hudson's trip to Paris, and suddenly it was everywhere. I couldn't pick up a newspaper or turn on the TV without learning more than I wanted to know. Hysteria swept the nation, and parents took to the streets to keep children with AIDS out of school. And so I began to feel the fear. Like every gay man who participated in the party of the Seventies, I check my skin for lesions after each shower and worry about every unexplained cough.

The fear is not just that I may become one of the statistics myself, but that I will become a pariah. Eager for justice, I have come out of the closet at the school on Staten Island where I teach. I am known to belong to a risk group. Will my health insurance be threatened? Would my colleagues maintain their liberalism if it meant that their insurance rates would go up to protect me? Will some parent insist that I am a danger to his or her child? Am I, in fact, a walking time bomb? Unwilling to volunteer my name for some quarantine list, I have not been tested for HIV antibodies, so I do not know for sure, but I behave as if I am infectious.

Last semester, I felt leery about coming out to my classes, although I had been doing it for years. It no longer seemed to be a social or political statement, but a medical one. Then I found my students giggling at something in class, which turned out to be a safe-sex leaflet: two stick figures performing anal intercourse in a circle with a slash mark through it, labeled "Ban AIDS." I came out to them that week. "There is nothing funny about AIDS," I told them. "We are not stick figures. We are real people." They sobered up fast enough, but I wonder how long their compassion will last.

I emerge from the dark cattle car, momentarily blinded by the new light. People around me are beginning to run wildly along the railroad tracks. Then I hear the sound of gunfire behind us, and I begin to run with them. We are wearing pink triangles, but I realize that they are shooting at us because we are Jews.

17

There are times when *Gone With the Wind* fails me. I grew up with tales of the Holocaust, and I invest much time in trying to understand its message about human nature, so it is small wonder that I found myself sitting through nine hours of the documentary *Shoah* (Hebrew for annihilation) a few months ago, listening to account after account of the unimaginable atrocities that are the stuff of human history.

Raul Hilberg, a Holocaust scholar, appears in the film. He sums up the history of Jewish persecution:

> . . . From the Fourth Century . . . the missionaries of Christianity had said in effect to the Jews: "You may not live among us as Jews." The secular rulers who followed them from the Middle Ages then decided: "You may not live among us," and the Nazis finally decreed, "You may not live." . . . And the "final solution," you see, is really final, because people who are converted can yet be Jews in secret, people who are expelled can yet return. But people who are dead will not reappear.

For centuries we have heard from the heterosexual majority, "You may not live among us as homosexuals," and the closet was our means of survival until we could tolerate it no longer. Are we now hearing, "You may not live among us," in the form of the threatened compulsory HIV testing and quarantine that several states are actively considering as law? Does it take much imagination to hear in the wind, "You may not live?"

For years we have been hearing of parallels between gays and Jews. Both groups are aliens in the countries of their birth, accused of disloyalty. Both bear stigmas as dangers to the culture at large—especially to its children, whom Jews were accused of sacrificing and gays of molesting. Both are accused of "bad blood." Immigration has been restricted for both. All these comparisons have been drawn before, but each year the list of parallels grows. This year, we are discussing tattoos, and official markers, perhaps health cards, comparable to yellow stars or passports stamped *J*. Jewish counsels (*Judenräte*) policed the Jewish community; gay "sex police" are already at work in Florida, enforcing safe-sex practices. Jews were told that resettlement would benefit them; gays are assured that compulsory testing for viral antibodies and quarantine would be in the public's best interest—nothing personal. Jewish businesses were closed; gay bathhouses are closing. Demagogues openly assaulted Jews and dehumanized them into caricatures in the controlled German press; gays are openly assaulted and robbed of their humanity in America's free press.

The Nazis waited until the Jews were too debilitated from hunger and disorientation to resist before rounding them up. Is someone waiting until we are sufficiently debilitated from disease? Will there be a "final solution" for American gays as there was for German gays and Jews? Will someone tell us the shower is only for "disinfection" and hand us bars of stone instead of soap? I cannot always distinguish between fear and foresight, but I know that humanity is capable of the worst as well as the best. Not even America would take in the desperate Jews of Europe when they tried to escape. What country would take in potential carriers of a deadly virus? There is nowhere to flee.

(The Siege of Atlanta brings bombshells into the heart of town. Scarlett arrives home to find her aunt preparing to flee.)

AUNT PITTY: "I can't bear it. Those cannonballs right in my ear . . . I may be a coward, but oh dear, Yankees in Georgia! How did they ever get in? . . . Uncle Peter, my smelling salts!"

(Scarlett, of course, stays through the chaos to help Melanie have her baby, but finally Scarlett, too, must flee. Rhett brings a carriage to rescue her.)

SCARLETT: "Wait! I forgot to lock the door." *(He laughs.)* "What are you laughing at?"

RHETT: "At you, locking the Yankees out."

Against such a background, it takes much of my energy to be even slightly helpful to Malcolm and my other friends. My lover and I gave a party to welcome Malcolm and Frank back to town, where they came so that they could be near their friends. Parties have their awkward moments these days. I find myself trying not to stare at someone's KS lesions, or listening to someone else's anger because a person with AIDS has greeted her with a kiss on the lips.

This party went reasonably well. David, a singer who now heads the National Persons With AIDS Coalition, was present, and another friend, Robert, was visiting from across the country, possibly for the last time. He'd lost his hair from the chemotherapy used to treat his lymph cancer, and his arm was becoming paralyzed so that he couldn't tie his shoes or zip his fly without help. If it was hard for me to look at him, it was twice as hard for Malcolm, who spent much of the time away from the crowd, musing on subjects such as whether it's worth saving receipts if one isn't sure that he will live to file an income tax return. "They've taken my future away," he said. I nodded silently, trying to understand what he was feeling, fishing for some inane encouragement to offer. The next day, Malcolm asked if I would be willing to help him die if the suffering became too bad.

A few days later, a friend of Malcolm's called to say that his brother Gordon was in a coma and had only a few days left. He wanted to know if it was wise to tell Malcolm. I ended up bringing the news to him, carefully waiting until he was in his kitchen, so that Frank, who was ill in the next room, would not hear and get upset. History was growing hard for them. They had begun to avoid the newspapers. Malcolm began to weep when I told him that Gordon was dying. He told me that only the day before, David, the singer, had told him of another mutual friend who'd just died. "Where will it end?" he asked. I did not answer.

At the end of the week, we sat together at Gordon's funeral. My lover, Larry, was at my side, but it was Malcolm's hand I was holding. The eulogy was a passage from Seneca: "He that has lost a friend has more cause for joy that he once had him than of grief that he is taken away." Malcolm and I looked into each other's tearful eyes, and we both knew that we were crying as much for the death that threatens to end our fifteen years of love as we were mourning for those already gone.

My frustration is mounting. I have dialed the number again and again but I cannot get the telephone at the other end to ring. Stubbornly refusing to yield, I keep dialing. There is never a response.

Only when I wake do I remember that the friend I was calling had died.

We are not the carefree Peter Pans we once were. We are aging before our time. When we meet old friends in the street, we remember to be glad they are still with us. Our conversation sounds much like my grandfather's did when he was in his eighties. "Did you hear that Charles died?" (We all read the obituary pages.) "Terrible, he was a good man." "I remember how he loved to dance." "It was a nice funeral." "George is ill." "Oh, no. When will it end?" "And you? How are you feeling?" "I'm okay. The doctor says it's just a cold." "Keep well." "You, too."

Sometimes in the midst of pain, the mind wanders back to a happier time. The moon hung low over Fire Island as we wound down our hours of disco. On mescaline, everything was more than real, and magic was in the air under a sky brilliant with stars. Wiping the dance sweat from our brows, we headed into the woods, guided by white painted tree stumps and the sound of the surf beyond the dunes. There we met as shadows, kissing flesh to flesh, mouth to cock and cock to ass, laughing like the pixies we were, sharing our orgiastic joy, shooting great jets of semen into the night with glee, drinking in one another's essence. We were all one man there—one body, one spirit—until the majestic sun arose, and we dwindled our way to sleep, resting for the next night's frolic.

(It is several years after the war. Scarlett enters the lumber mill where Ashley is working. Though she looks no older, her face is perceptibly hardened and her whole bearing more mature. They begin to reminisce.)

ASHLEY: *". . .* I'll always be haunted by the memory of a charm and beauty that are gone forever . . . oh, the lazy days and warm still country twilights! . . . The golden warmth and security of those days!"

SCARLETT *(tears in her eyes)*: "Don't look back, Ashley! Don't look back! It drags at your heart till you can't do anything but look back!"

Sixteen years ago, I came out of the closet and onto the stage of gay politics. Within a few short months, I went from a life of timidity and isolation and blackmail threats to a life of courage and community and confrontation as the secretary and then the vice-president of the Gay Activists Alliance, at that time the largest gay civil rights organization in the East. I took to the streets, the press, and the airwaves to proclaim that I was gay and to demand equality.

Jim Owles and I took the first draft of GAA's gay civil rights bill to New York City Councilman Eldon Clingon in 1970, and the long, well-chronicled struggle for my city's recognition of my civil rights began. In the course of it, I would be arrested and tried, praised for my courage and damned for my "perversion." I was so convinced of the justice of our cause that it came as a genuine surprise to me that America didn't open her arms immediately and take us to her national bosom. I learned that the fight for equality would be long and hard, but at least my own life had been permanently changed. I had new friends, new values, and new self-confidence.

Eventually, my ardor for political meetings waned. I kept active by writing, and I became involved in gay groups on an ad hoc basis, joining the Gay Academic Union one year and the Christopher Street Liberation Day Committee to arrange the annual march down Fifth Avenue another. But I kept my friends, my values, and my confidence that I was a worthwhile human being.

Then came the AIDS backlash and the fear. Last fall saw Louis Welch saying on the radio, "Shoot the queers!" and Paul Cameron on TV calling openly for our extermination. The Republican candidate for New York mayor that season endorsed the forced closing of all baths and bars and compulsory testing for antibodies, announcing, "The AIDS virus has no civil rights." Great humanitarians all.

I am searching through the cobwebs and rubble for my friends, so that we can celebrate the end of the world together. The lights flicker and go dim. I discover a dusty bottle of champagne, vintage unknown, so the party can begin as soon as I find the others. Where are they?

The most valuable lesson in 1970 had been that I was not alone. Sharing my plight and my struggle with others like me had given me the strength to do more than I knew I was capable of. I learned the same lesson in 1985. When I heard that a political meeting was being called, I left work early to get there on time. A small group of concerned people rapidly grew into the Gay and Lesbian Alliance Against Defamation (GLAAD), and I became its secretary.

Within weeks, we called our first town meeting to discuss our hopes and fears—seven hundred people who felt the same way I did showed up! Soon we were all confronting the *New York Post*, demanding an end to its blatant fag-baiting and piling rags on its doorstep to show its editors what their newspaper really is. What the *Post* thinks is less important than the anger we unleashed. Fear turned to rage, and rage soon became determination. Now GLAAD is organized to respond to homophobia in the media and government with letters and phone calls, negotiations and demonstrations. Maybe we're not totally safe from an uncertain future, but at least we're together, and that helps immeasurably in the fight against fear. Best of all, the people who gained experience sixteen years ago are able to share it with a new generation of activists and to see their ideas continue and grow.

Hope for the future may ease the fear, but it does not ease the pain. While Malcolm was away on a trip, I got word that Frank was gravely ill. He had flown to the Northwest, his favorite place, and that meant frantic phone calls first to the hospital, then halfway around the globe to find Malcolm. He rushed to Frank's side immediately, but he didn't arrive in time, and he was wracked with guilt because of it.

His final glimpse of Frank was of a corpse wrapped in plastic in a drawer in the morgue. He stayed a few days and supervised Frank's cremation and strewed Frank's ashes, flying back the same day. He took a small canister from his luggage and opened it to show me its contents. Small shards of bright white bone nestled together in it. "I saved some of Frank's ashes," he said. I felt embarrassed at this final intimacy with Frank, as if I had unexpectedly seen my grandmother naked, but I felt there was something sacred about the contents of the canister. Malcolm kept picking at his scalp. I asked if he was having some problem. "It's Frank's ashes," he said. "It was very windy while we were strewing them, and I didn't have a chance to take a shower."

Filip Müller was a *Sonderkommando*, one of the inmates who emptied the gas chambers at Auschwitz. In *Shoah*, he tells what he saw there.

People fell out like blocks of stone, like rocks falling out of a truck. . . . The people were battered. They struggled and fought in the darkness. They were covered in excrement, in blood, from ears and noses. One also sometimes saw that the people lying on the ground, because of the pressure of the others, were unrecognizable. . . . Every day we saw thousands and thousands of innocent people disappear up the chimney. With our own eyes, we could truly fathom what it means to be a human being. There they came, men, women, children, all innocent. They suddenly vanished, and the world said nothing! We felt abandoned. By the world, by humanity. But the situation taught us fully what the possibility of survival meant. For we could gauge the infinite value of human life. And we were convinced that hope lingers in man as long as he lives. Where there's life, hope must never be relinquished. That's why we struggled through our lives of hardship, day after day, week after week, month after month, year after year, hoping against hope to survive, to escape that hell.

If you wait long enough, things seem to come full circle. The AIDS crisis has brought homophobes of every stripe out of the woodwork, and their fulminations against us have inadvertently helped to make some decent people aware of the real threats faced by the gay community and of the need for legislation to protect us.

When New York City's gay rights bill, Intro 2, surfaced once again in the city council, our enemies called us abominations and sinners, negative role models and child molesters, trying to impose their primitive values on our lives. While Pope John Paul II counsels his priests to refrain from involvement in secular affairs, Cardinal O'Connor shamelessly lobbies with legislators and politicizes his pulpit.

But I am most appalled at the Orthodox Jews, who see no relationship between their right to be different and mine, who wear skullcaps and side curls to display their religious beliefs and tell me I am flaunting my private life, who hear no echoes of the Holocaust in the talk of tattooing gay forearms. What the *Sonderkommandos* of Auschwitz learned at such a high price is completely lost on them. If they ran this city, they would probably follow the biblical injunction to stone homosexuals to death and feel sanctimonious about it. They turned their backs on Mayor Koch as he spoke in support of gay rights, but it is they who are alone, not we.

Waiting near the radio for the city council's vote to be broadcast, I thought of how some survivor of the Holocaust might have felt waiting for the results of the UN vote on the partition of Israel as an independent state. There was a mixture of gladness and guilt that I had lived to see it while others I knew had not. Before I left the closet in 1970, I was so intimidated by ignorance and hatred that I tried to kill myself twice, but I survived to see the best years of my life. Once again, the ignorance and hatred surround me, but Intro 2 gives me some hope that if I can endure through this dark time, something better may follow.

Who knows? If we work at it, we might win still more, perhaps even the right to marry and the legal, social, and economic advantages that come with it. Whatever we achieve, we must not let the next generation become complacent and take these treasures for granted, or they will be lost to us again.

As I stood with my lover and Malcolm amidst the throng in Sheridan Square, surrounded by old friends from GAA and new friends from GLAAD, celebrating the passage of the law for which we had all fought so long and hard, I felt a quiet pride. (I did some leaping and whooping, too.) We have made it the hard way, and we will have to fight to preserve what little we have gained. Some of us will not survive to see the future, but those of us who do must learn, as Filip Müller did, "the infinite value of human life." Our enemies foolishly turn their backs on us and fail to appreciate how much we have to give, but their rejection only makes us stronger and more self-reliant.

SCARLETT: "But, Rhett, if you go what shall I do? Where shall I go?"

RHETT: "Frankly, my dear, I don't give a damn!"

(After Rhett has gone, Scarlett sits on her staircase to ponder her future. A beautiful smile of hope crosses her face as the realization comes to her that she still has Tara. . . . She lifts her chin higher. We see the stuff of which Scarlett O'Hara is made, and we thrill with the knowledge that she won't be defeated for long.)

SCARLETT: "After all, tomorrow is another day!"

Wandering the Woods in a
Season of Death

ALLAN TROXLER

Durham, North Carolina
March 26, 1983

Dear Leo,

Went to the woods the other afternoon. Thought you might like a report—your man on assignment in the Eastern hardwood forest.

Taking the wide path off Whitfield Road, first thing you pass leggy jack pines tangled with honeysuckle. Within memory, this was cornfields and tobacco. No old growth, to speak of.

Over the last few years since I came back, I've pondered the state of the Piedmont woodlands some. It's been a process of unlearning a Sierra Club book vision of nature. One sweaty afternoon late last spring, I stretched on the cool clay bank of Cane Creek, watched the light glowing through the dense vines, breathed the dank creek smell, and half-listened to several friends from Vermont nattering about the poison ivy and the bugs. I studied the opalescent interior of a freshwater clam shell and just smiled.

I went walking out in Duke Forest in the spring, my eyes and ears informed by the dying of a friend. I discovered, in the order of things

27

*there, intimations of my own death, and of yours—the tree trunk
resting on the slope, the water's timeless sounds. There was reas-
surance to this wandering through the woods's gradual changes and
through seasons. For some, though, there is the forest fire, or the
hunter.*

I caught myself hurrying on past the honeysuckle and scrub
pine the other day, partly because it was getting late and I
wanted to find things to report to you, and partly because of
those old prejudices. Then I got to thinking of the honeysuckle's beneficient smell—in my North Carolina *grand cru*,
along with the wood thrush's song, lightning bugs, thun-
derstorms, muscadines, rabbit tobacco, and winter sunsets. I
slowed down. What right have I, a left-handed Southern
queer, to snub a fellow weed? So pausing to respect the honeysuckle, I wish to report that its exuberant vines were span-
gled with tiny new leaves.

In the blowing snow the next day, I saw a pear tree in full
bloom and couldn't tell where the flowers ended and the snow
began.

*Leo and I came to share our love for the woods of childhood—his in
Alabama and Virginia, mine in North Carolina—when we were in
college together. Years later, our paths converged in the rough moun-
tains of southern Oregon. He had heard of Wolf Creek, where Carl
and I and our friends lived, and he sought us out.*

*Leo was wrestling, such as he ever did anything head-on, with the
problem of being gay and being a doctor. He had recently finished med
school and was just beginning to come out. In Oregon, we walked
under the madrones and Doug firs, and out on the slopes where the
ceanothus bloomed deep sky-blue, and talked.*

*He told me of his doctor mother and his lawyer father; of how all
along he had met their expectations, more or less; of the placid course
of his life until recently.*

Generally, when Leo approached passion over anything, the lower half of his face would get amused, the upper half mildly distressed, his voice would sort of crack and give out and, directly, the intensity would pass. But in Wolf Creek this time his anguish lingered. He stayed with us for several months, fretting.

Looking down on a buckeye sapling, I was powerfully taken by the geometry of the ruddy new leaves, stems going off at right angles, then leafing out in fives, deeply ribbed, ready to unfurl and spread.

Why is order in nature so exciting? Crystals, skeletons, shells—why this hankering for symmetry? I assume it's not an exclusively human tropism. Recently, I noticed a wasp nest in a sourwood tree. Surely the wasps would not have settled for less-regular cells. Honeybees refuse machine-made comb when the hexagons are off the least bit. And the Greenpeace people report that whales and dolphins will follow along for miles listening, rapt, to Mozart. There you have it, whatever it is.

Finally, Leo decided to move to San Francisco, where he found work with a group of gay doctors. I remember climbing the hills in Buena Vista park with him, up behind his office, and comparing the rhododendrons there with those back East. For all the wonders of the Northwest coast, we both longed for the woods back home. "Eastern hardwood forest" became code between us, a metaphor for Home, from which we were in exile, trying to become ourselves.

In the dwindling light down by the creek, a pale cocoon hung from a twig. I'll keep an eye on it. The steely water shone against the dark hills. Upstream the rocks rattled against each other.

* * *

In 1979, I moved back to North Carolina to hazard being openly gay in a place I loved after a fashion, and which I understood. (Oregon is closer to Japan than to Europe and the dogwoods there have five petals.) On my last trip down to San Francisco, there were posters everywhere protesting the fate of Joann Little and the Wilmington 10. I needed to get on home.

Years passed, Leo and I lost touch, and then I heard through a college friend that Leo had AIDS. The opportunistic infection was severe meningitis. He could neither talk nor see. He had a reservoir for drugs implanted in his skull.

I wanted to communicate somehow, yet I didn't want to taunt him with the details of my daily life. I decided on a journal, of sorts, from our Eastern hardwood forest. Hickory and trout lily could be our vocabulary. Possum and star.

April 18

Dear Leo,

Since I last wrote, late winter has turned to high spring, practically. Bare branch to leaf, bud to seedpod. Rest, stir, swell, split, sprout, rise, spread, bloom, fruit, seed, droop, shed, rot, rest. It all keeps changing; except for water, light, and air, which are pretty constant, aren't they? Or rather they don't change like organisms change. I guess.

In a way, though, the vast spectrum of events attendant upon the coming and going of light every day is like an organism; still dark, first stirring, sap rising, breath quickening, chirping, humming, speaking, light to sugar, air to Co_2, land warming, wind shifting, and so on. And isn't a pond or creek a body in some animate sense? Breathing, generating, waking, sleeping.

Oh, Leo. Such medieval animism. My mind has gone to seed. Well, to begin. The sun is still up and the light which suffuses the intricate infinity of pale-gray trunks and branches tempts me to rise and float among them creekward. Sometime I float in my dreams. Aside from feeling lifted up by my heart and my lungs, I especially enjoy the state of being untouched—free of floor, chair, bed, table—moving among things unencumbered. Floating outdoors, however, is another matter. Uncontained, I rise higher and faster, and invariably, when landscapes have dwindled to tiny patterns, I lose it and hurtle earthward. But in the pellucid woods this afternoon, with a ceiling of branches, floating is safe. I believe tonight will be the full moon.

On my walks, I got to thinking about what we choose to perceive, and how. It's such a temptation, to which I often succumb, to celebrate the perky signs of life without paying attention to quieter, more extended processes. When the lavender-crested irises spangle the slope by the creek, who notices the fallen beech leaves there, pale and curved, damp, darkening, and then letting go into earth? And when one does take the time to study those subtler events (the returning, from the going forth), where are the words to describe them positively, or at least with neutrality? Our words are hobbled by our fear of dying.

As I watched and listened for things that spoke to Leo's waning, to his coming stillness, I reckon I was loosening my own fatuous grip on immortality a little.

One afternoon, an air raid siren tore through the quietness. "So this is it. He's gone and done it." Half-seriously, I thought to lie down in the leaves and wait for destruction to sweep through the trees. The only regret I could imagine was not being with those I love most. Otherwise, my own death seemed brother to the empty wasp nest, the bleached box turtle shell, the lichen on the rocks, and the soughing water.

Then I remembered the volunteer fire department nearby.

*   *   *

In the dusk, two small white clouds hang over the creek; a long bleached bone lies on the bank. A shad tree in bloom; a cedar skeleton.

Tennis shoes on firm sand rippled by the winter floods. Such elating closeness with earth, suddenly after calbering downhill through the noisy leaves. Roots/veins/sinews stretch across the path. I slow to stroke a muscular ironwood trunk. A comely young man lopes up the path out of the dark—"H'lo" "H'lo"— and passes. My ears pound.

Then I hurry downstream to find the cocoon. I can barely see. Have I gone too far? I backtrack. No. Must be farther on. Downstream again. Where the creek foams noisily, it is hanging out over the water, suspended on a thin ligature from its branch. Ovoid, rough. Waiting.

I hadn't expected Leo to respond, I guess, but as the woods became opaque green and the heat settled in, I got out there for walks less and less, and eventually with no word from San Francisco, I stopped writing.

Early one morning before the air got feverish, I walked downstream to check on the cocoon. There was no sign of it ever having been there.

With fall and then winter, the epidemic moved in over our daily lives, with its low clouds and its chill. A friend in Durham was diagnosed. An acquaintance in Chapel Hill died. Several friends organized the N.C. Lesbian and Gay Health Project, and as part of that I began visiting a man over at the V.A. Hospital, who had moved back from San Francisco to be nearer his family out in Marion.

Talk didn't come readily for Michael and me. Often he would keep on staring at the TV, so I took to massaging his skinny legs and swollen feet, and then his rigid shoulders and his bruised face.

"Brings me flowers and rubs my legs," he explained to a new nurse in his soft mountain voice.

I didn't know if Leo was alive or dead. The reports of his meningitis had been so severe, I figured he was gone. Then word came that he was in D.C. He had rallied unexpectedly, as is the case with AIDS sometimes, and had come back East to see his folks. Things were fine and then suddenly they weren't and now he was in a fancy hospital up there.

May 7, 1984

Dear Carl [My partner/friend Carl had just gone to Europe for two months],

The time with Leo was pretty good. Like Michael, he's starved for touching. Says about the only contact he has now is with cold medical instruments and hypodermic needles. He's gaunt and weak but a good deal chattier than M. has become. Nothing much profound to our talk, but still it seemed important.

Being around his mother, a gracious woman who brings lilacs, bleeding hearts, and lily of the valley from their place in McLean, puts me in mind of *The Garden of the Finzi-Continis*, except these Jews are Southern.

Michael died on May the 16th. With Gail, his generous, feisty little sister, I watched his crusted lips opening and closing, slower, slower, and his unseeing eyes. "You stubborn bastard! You just won't die, will you?" She cried and laughed at the same time. The gaping mouth slacked and, finally, was still. Something in me felt like a bass getting ripped from a pond.

We held on to each other and wept.

May 19, D.C.

Dear Carl,

Leo sleeps now, drugged for the injection into the reservoir in his skull, coming shortly, that will make him extremely nauseated. Before he dozed off, he told the nurse he was afraid.

I see now why Whitman embraced the chance to nurse Civil War soldiers. Surely the democracy of death confirmed all the egalitarian effusion of *Leaves of Grass*. Here the waiting, the pain, the wasting away are familiar from Michael's ordeal at the V.A. The fuss about petty things, the erosion of civility. Although Leo still says "Thank you" after I massage his legs— a vestige of his rearing—mostly such differences fade and he and Michael, who clog-danced for nickels at the bus station as a boy, become brothers.

Last time I was up, Leo talked about how exciting the gay scene in SF was at first. A chance for him to be close to men he had been protected from growing up in the patrician burbs.

Now the doctor is injecting the drug into his head, which will incite vomiting.

Next day, Sunday

Bedside again. Leo's sleeping. With long hawk-beak nose and sunken cheeks, he looks like an unwrapped mummy, or the Danish bog man. Today there's a new IV hooked up, this time into his foot. Blood and sodium solution.

Yesterday his mother, who in spite of breeding is rattled by her son's ignominious demise, insisted that Tom and I drive out to McLean to visit. Now, looking at Leo, I see a good bit more than before. Their place is all vast lawns with grand plantings of azalea and boxwood. Huge oaks. Leo's mother was just coming up from the pool, in her bathrobe and espadrilles. I had thought her invitation might be a muted call for help, but as she led us from flower bed to flower bed, she seemed put upon and distracted. Here were rare azaleas. Here the enormous rhododendrons Leo had planted as a boy.

Leo's father stalked around in pajamas, growling at the Salvadoran yard boy, who had scattered the tools. No time, just a few gruff words, for his son's faggot friends. Small wonder Leo always seemed paralyzed—partly from waiting for the next silver platter to come around, and partly from the terror of a bitter, disappointed father.

So here I am, back watching the ruined scion sleep, crumpled among engulfing sheets and gown. A week ago, his Puerto Rican lover, Ramon, visited. He's young, working-class. Glad I wasn't a fly on the mansion wall for that.

Monday, May 21

Once Leo woke up yesterday, I helped him with his lunch and we talked a little. I asked him how he would rather this all have proceeded and immediately he said he wished he was back in California with his lover and friends.

I'm tempted to call the gay clinic in D.C. and inquire about folks to visit Leo. In the hall as I was leaving, I asked one of his nurses whether she knew of anybody visiting AIDS cases—they have five or six there. She looked confused and a tetch nonplussed and said she hadn't run into anyone. It made me value our Health Project work more, and to appreciate the warmth of some of the V.A. staff. I reckon those country club hospitals tend to be high tech and low empathy sometimes.

And so I part ways with Leo. Back in college, when he

would bake shortbread in the biology lab oven during all-night study jags, or when we luxuriated among the camellias in the snow-covered greenhouse, or wore our English country whites for dancing "Spring Garden" and "Step Stately," I would never have guessed that twenty years later I would mop up the diarrhea in which he lay, or stroke his stubbly, waxen face as he dozed in a drugged stupor.

July 20

Dear Carl,

Late Thursday night, I got a call from Ramon Santos, Leo's lover in SF. Leo died June 21. His family buried him quickly and notified none of his gay friends. For the last month, Leo couldn't, or wouldn't, talk. Ramon would call and talk to a silent void. He was going through Leo's papers and found the letters I wrote last spring. Funny to have such a forthright, emotional conversation in the middle of the night with a man I've never met.

It will be years and years before we understand the magnitude of this AIDS experience. I wonder that it might prove to be one of the major events of late twentieth-century culture. The minstrels become Greek chorus.

I was too shook up when we were done to go back to bed. I fetched ballpoint and pad, put on my sneakers, and drove out to the woods, to retrace the route I used to take and to comtemplate. The moon was full and the lightning bugs were out, but as I walked, the woods got darker and darker; I got all turned around and scared and I could only think about trying to find my way out. A storm was coming on. For a while, the lightning helped, then the rain set in and I got soaked.

Finding a path in leaves, on earth, is one thing in the dark. Groping along on jagged rocks in a downpour is another. I thought about how death is graceless—getting lost on terrain that was once familiar and then suddenly is strange and hostile. Maybe ten feet away, something gnawed loudly. Teeth on shell or tough wood or bone. A startling, private sound.

A few hours later, I ended up on Whitfield Road, somehow, standing shirtless in the rain, staring up at the sky, breathing deep.

September 12

Now Warren, Glen, and Philip have died, too.

In the woods, the thin, high songs of crickets merge with the wind in the trees, like a distant river. I process through this world of leaves, waving a dogwood branch to fend off spiderwebs and beggar's-lice.

I pass the shiny orange berries of the hearts a-bustin', hanging from their deep pink hulls; then the stiff brown seed heads of self-heal, or heal-all. After weeks of terrible heat, the morning is cool and gray. Down by the creek, a spike of cardinal flower glows blood red.

The Fear

ANDREW HOLLERAN

The Fear is of course unseemly—as most fear is. People behave at worst with demonic cruelty—at best oddly. Even among those who are good-hearted, the madness breaks out in small ways that bring friendships of long standing to an abrupt end. When the plague began and the television crews of certain TV stations refused to work on interviews with people with AIDS, I wanted to get their names, write them down, publish them on a list of cowards. When the parents in Queens picketed and refused to send their kids to school; when they kicked Ryan White out of class in Indiana; when people called in to ask if it was safe to ride the subway; when Pat Buchanan called for a quarantine of homosexuals; when they burned down the house in Arcadia, Florida, I felt a thrilling disgust, a contempt, an anger at the shrill, stupid, mean panic, the alacrity with which people are converted to lepers and the lepers cast out of the tribe, the fact that if Fear is contemptible, it is most contemptible in people who have no reason to fear.

Even within the homosexual community, however, there was despicable behavior: men who would not go to restaurants, hospital rooms, wakes, for fear that any contact with other homosexuals might be lethal. At dinner one night in San Francisco in 1982, a friend said, "There's a crack in the glass," after I'd taken a sip of his lover's wine, and took the glass back to the kitchen to replace it—a reaction so swift it took me a moment to realize there was no crack in the glass; the problem was my lips' touching it—homosexual lips, from New York: the kiss of death. I was furious then, but the behavior no longer surprises me. AIDS, after all, belongs to the Age of Anxiety. My friend was a germophobe to begin with, who, though homosexual himself, after five years in San Francisco, had come to loathe homosexuals. The idea that they could now kill him, or his lover, fit in. AIDS fed on his free-floating anxiety about the rest of modern life: the fertilizers, pesticides, toxic wastes, additives in food, processing of food, steroids given cattle, salmonella in chickens, killer bees moving up from Brazil, Mediterranean fruit fly, poisoned water, lead in our pipes, radon in our homes, asbestos in our high schools, danger of cigarette smoke, mercury in tuna, auto emissions in the air, Filipinos on the bus, Mexicans sneaking across the border. The society that could make sugar sinister was ready, it would seem, to panic over AIDS, so that when Russia put out the disinformation in its official press that AIDS was the work of a germ-warfare laboratory run by the Pentagon, it was only repeating a charge made by homosexuals convinced that AIDS is a right-wing program to eradicate queers.

God only knows what AIDS will turn out to be, years and years from now—perhaps, in 2005, "Sixty Minutes" will reveal it *was* a CIA foul-up. But this general panic, this unease, this sense that the world is out of control and too intimately connected, is not *all* the Fear is among homosexuals. The Fear among homosexuals is personal, physical, and real. It is easy enough to dismiss the idea that the CIA set out to exterminate homosexuals; it is not easy to dismiss the fact that—having lived in New York during the seventies as a gay man—one can reasonably expect to have been infected. "We've all been exposed," a friend said to me in 1981 on the sidewalk one evening before going off to Switzerland to have his blood recycled—when "exposed" was still the word to spare the feelings of those who were, someone finally pointed out, "infected." The idea—that everyone had been swimming in the same sea—made little impression on us at the time; nor did I grasp the implications—because then the plague was still so new, and its victims so (relatively) few, that most homosexuals could still come up with a list of forty to fifty things to distinguish their past, their habits, from those of the men they knew who had it. Now, five years later, that list in is shreds; one by one, those distinguishing features or habits have been taken away, and the plague reveals itself as something infinitely larger, more various, more random, than was suspected at the start—as common as the flu—indeed, the thing the doctors are predicting a repeat of: the Spanish influenza following World War I.

Predictions like these, above all, intensify the Fear, to the point that one tenses when a news story comes on the evening news about AIDS—and wonders: What new sadistic detail? What new insoluble problem? One looks away when the word is in the newspaper headline and turns to the comics instead. One hopes the phone will not ring with news of yet another friend diagnosed, because one can always trace a flare-up of the Fear—an AIDS anxiety attack: that period when you are certain you have It, and begin making plans for your demise—to some piece of news, or several, that came through the television or the telephone. Sometimes they are so numerous, and all at once, that you are undone—like the man walking down the boardwalk on Fire Island with a friend one evening on their way to dance, who, after a quiet conversation at dinner, suddenly threw himself down on the ground and began screaming: "We're all going to die, we're all going to die!" He did. Sometimes it hits like that. It appears in the midst of the most ordinary circumstances—like the man on that same beach, who in the middle of a cloudless summer afternoon turned to my friend and said: "What is the point of going on?" ("To bear witness," my friend responded.) The Fear is there all the time, but it comes in surges, like electricity—activated, triggered, almost always by specific bad news.

The media are full of bad news, of course—the stories of breakthroughs, of discoveries, of new drugs seem to have subsided now into a sea of disappointment. They do not sound the note of relief and hope and exultation they once did—that dream that one evening you would be brushing your teeth, and your roommate, watching the news in the living room, would shout: "It's over!" and you would run down the hall and hear the Armistice declared. Instead, the media carry the *pronunciamientos* of the Harvard School of Public Health, the World Health Organization, dire beyond our wildest nightmares: What began as a strange disease ten or twelve homosexuals in New York had contracted becomes the Black Death. Of course, journalists, as Schopenhauer said, are professional alarmists, and have only fulfilled their usual role: scaring their readers. They are scaring them so that the readers will protect themselves, of course; they are at the same time inducing despair in those already infected. There's the dilemma: They're all watching the same TV, reading the same newspapers.

After a while, the Fear is so ugly you feel like someone at a dinner party whose fellow guests are being taken outside and shot as you concentrate politely on your salad. There is the school of thought that says the Fear is a form of stress, and stress enhances the virus. Like the man so afraid of muggers he somehow draws them to him, the Fear is said to make itself come true, by those who believe in mind control. As a friend of mine (so fearful of the disease he refused to have sex for four years) said, "I got everything I resisted." So one becomes fearful even of the Fear. The Fear can be so wearing, so depressing, so constant that a friend who learned he had AIDS said, on hearing the diagnosis, "Well, it's a lot better than worrying about it."

He also said, "I wasn't doing anything anyone else wasn't." Which explains the Fear more succinctly than anything else:

Tens of thousands were doing the same thing in the Seventies. Why, then, should some get sick and not others? Isn't it logical to expect everyone will, eventually? The Fear is so strong it causes people to change cities, to rewrite their pasts in order to imagine they were doing less than everyone else; because the most unnerving thing about the plague is its location in the Past, the Time allotted to it.

Were AIDS a disease which, once contracted, brought death within forty-eight hours of exposure, it would be a far more easily avoided illness—but because it is not—because it is invisible, unknown, for such a long period of time, because it is something people got before they even knew it existed (with each passing year, the Time Lag gets longer), the Fear of AIDS is limitless. Who has not had sex within the last seven years— once? (The nun in San Francisco who got AIDS from a blood transfusion given her during an operation to set her broken leg, and died, her superiors said, without anger or bitterness.) (The babies who get it in the womb.) There's a memory—of an evening, an incident—to justify every Fear. And nothing exists that will guarantee the fearful that even if they are functioning now, they will not get caught in the future. The phrase that keeps running through the fearful mind is: Everyone was healthy before he got sick. One has to have two programs, two sets of responses, ready at all times: (a) Life, (b) Death. The switch from one category to the other can come at any moment, in the most casual way. At the dentist's, or putting on your sock. Did that shin bruise a little too easily? Is that a new mole? Is the sinus condition that won't go away just a sinus condition? Do you feel a bit woozy standing at the kitchen sink? Do you want to lie down? Is the Fear making you woozy, or the virus? Have you had too many colds this past spring to be just colds? Thus the hyperconsciousness of the body begins. Your body—which you have tended, been proud of—is something you begin to view with suspicion, mistrust. Your body is someone you came to a party with and you'd like to ditch, only you promised to drive him home. Your body is a house—there's a thief inside it who wants to rob you of everything. Your body could be harboring It, even as you go about your business. This keeps you on edge. You stop, for instance, looking in mirrors. Or at your body in the shower—because the skin, all of a sudden, seems as vast as Russia: a huge terrain, a monumental wall, on which tiny handwriting may suddenly appear. The gums, the tongue, the face, the foot, the forearm, the leg: *billions* of cells waiting to go wrong. Because you read that sunburn depresses the immune system, you no longer go out in the sun. You stay in the house—as if already an invalid—you cancel all thoughts of traveling in airplanes because you heard flights can trigger the pneumonia and because you want to be home when it happens, not in some hotel room in Japan or San Diego.

And so the Fear constricts Life. It suffocates, till one evening its prey snaps—gets in the car and drives to the rest stop, or bar, or baths to meet another human being; and has sex. Sometimes has sex; sometimes just talks about the Fear, because a conversation about the danger of sex sometimes replaces sex itself. The Fear is a god to which offerings must be made before sex can commence. Sometimes it refuses the offering. If it does not, it takes its share of the harvest afterward. Sex serves the Fear more slavishly than anything. Even safe sex leads to the question: Why was I even doing something that *required* condoms? The aftermath of sex is fear *and* loathing. AIDS is a national program of aversion therapy. Sex and terror are twins. Death is a hunk, a gorgeous penis. And fear is self-centered, is above all personal, and you vent your terror before you realize how insensitive this is. One day you spill out your fears about the sex you had to a friend who—you realize too late—has had AIDS for a couple of years now. He has lived with his own fear for two years. Your friend merely listens calmly, says what you did does not seem unsafe, and then remarks: "What I'm getting from what you've been saying is that you're still afraid."

Of course, you want to reply, *of course* I'm still afraid! "But you have no reason to be," he says, from the height, the eminence of his own fear, digested, lived with, incorporated into his own life by now. "If you don't have it now, you won't." (Your other friend has told you, "The doctors think we're about to see a second wave of cases, the ones who contracted it in 1981.") Going home on the subway, your fear takes the form of superstition: He should never have said that! He himself had said (a remark you've never forgotten) that he was diagnosed just at the point when—after three years of abstinence—he thought he had escaped. It's the Time Lag, of course, the petri dish in which the Fear thrives. Of course, you are afraid; every male homosexual who lived in New York during the Seventies is scared shitless. And a bit unstable, withdrawn, and crazy. The tactlessness of venting your fear to a friend who already has been diagnosed is symptomatic of this behavior. People who are afraid are seldom as considerate as those who are unafraid. The ironic thing about my last visit to New York was that the two men I knew who have AIDS were cheerful, calm, gracious, well behaved. Those who did not were nervous wrecks: depressed, irritable, isolated, withdrawn, unwilling to go out at night, in bed by ten under a blanket, with terror and a VCR. The Fear is not fun to live with, though when shared, it can produce occasional, hysterical laughter. The laughter vanishes, however, the moment you leave the apartment building and find yourself alone on the street. Falls right off your face as you slip instantly back into the mood you were in before you went to visit your friend. The Fear breeds depression. The depression breeds anger. (Not to mention the anger of people who have it toward those who don't. Why me? Why should *he* escape?) Friendships come to an end over incidents which would have been jokes before. People withdraw from each other so they don't have to go through the suffering of each other's illness. People behave illogically: One night a friend refuses to eat from a buffet commemorating a dead dancer because so many of the other guests have AIDS ("They shouldn't have served finger food."), but he leaves the wake with a young handsome Brazilian who presumably doesn't, goes home and has sex. We all have an explanation for our private decisions, our choices of what we will do and what we won't; we all have a rationale for our superstitions. Most of it *is* superstition, because that is what the Fear produces and always has. Some of it is just muddled thinking, like the nightclub patrons in Miami who said they did not worry about AIDS there because it cost ten dollars to get in. And some of it is perfectly rational, like that which convinces people they should not take the Test because they would rather not live with the knowledge they have antibodies to the virus. (Today, the news announces a home test that will tell you in three minutes if you do, or don't; not much time for counseling!)

The Test is the most concentrated form of the Fear that there is—which is why people are advised not to take it if they think they will have trouble handling the results. Why should we know? The fact is things are happening in our bodies, our blood, all the time we know nothing of; the hole in the dyke of our immune systems may appear at any moment, and is always invisible, silent, unadvertised.

When does a person begin to develop cancer? When does a tumor start to grow? When does the wall of the heart begin to weaken? Do you want to know? With AIDS, there is presumably something in hiding, in the brain, the tissues, waiting for some moment to begin its incredibly fast and protean reproduction. It may be waiting—or reproducing—as I type this. This is the Fear that is finally selfish. That is perhaps worse in the imagining than in the reality. This is what makes you think: I must know, I can't bear this, I'll take the Test. So you drive over one hot afternoon to do it, thinking of the letter from a woman whose nephew just died at home of AIDS: "Tony even tested Negative two months before he died." What fun. You feel as if you are driving not toward the county health department but the Day of Judgment. In my right hand, I give you Life, in my left, Death. What will you do, the voice asks, when you find out? How will you live? How do people with AIDS drive the car, fall asleep at night, face the neighbors, deal with solitude? The stupendous cruelty of this disease crashes in upon you. And so you bargain with God. You apologize, and make vows. Ask, How could this have happened? How could I have reached this point? Where did I make the turn that got me on *this* road? Every test you have ever taken, written or oral—the book reports; the thesis examinations; the spelling bees; those afternoons walking home from school as far as you could before turning the page of your test to see the grade, on a corner where no one could see your reaction; the day you got drafted; the day you found out whether you were going to Vietnam—all pale, or come back, in one single concentrated tsunami of terror at this moment.

In eighteenth-century Connecticut, Jonathan Edwards preached a sermon called "Sinners in the Hands of an Angry God," which was so terrifying that women in the congregation fainted. Some things never change. The Fear, like the sermon, feeds on the Imagination. And the moment you know someone who faces this disease daily with composure, calm, humor, and his or her own personality intact, you realize how deforming, how demeaning, how subject to the worst instincts Fear is.

A Letter Home on Pride Day

ALLAN TROXLER

Salem, New York
Saturday, June 28, 1986

Dear Friends,

Right now many of you are marching down Ninth Street, with posters aloft and banners flapping. I wish I could be there, but since I can't, here are some thoughts for the day, mostly about our neighbors on Vale Street, in East Durham. We can't get to where we're going as gay people without help, so today I'd like to tell you about Hannah Hartel, Louise Petty, and John Thomas Satterfield. And to say "Thank you."

Mrs. Hartel was born down east in Onslow County, eighty-six years ago. Her people wrestled a living from land where alligators wandered through the cornfields and where disease and death worked right alongside of you. When my friend Carl and I first moved to Vale Street, Mrs. Hartel would come by, peering out shyly from the shade of her big sunbonnet, to offer us cuttings for our garden. We despaired of ever getting to know her since she was stone-deaf, it seemed, and she refused to come in, as it wasn't proper for a lady to visit men unaccompanied, she said. But now as I think about it, more likely it was she wouldn't have anywhere to spit her tobacco juice.

By and by, we listened to lugubrious monologues about her

husband, who had been an alcoholic, and how she had buried all her sons, also from drink, except for her last, who was in prison again. But then they let him out, since he was pretty far gone from cancer and wanted to come home to die. And that's how we really got to know Mrs. Hartel.

One night, she called for one of us to go after medicine and when I got down there with it, he was dying. A few days later, Carl and I pieced together our most respectable clothes and walked to Hudson's funeral home to be pallbearers for Willie Edward.

After that, Mrs. Hartel took to inviting us for Sunday dinner, along with Robert, the cigar-chomping saw-sharpener, and Randy, the Hell's Angel. She called us her "boys." I would usually take a mason jar full of flowers and sometimes I'd bake a pie or something. As we grew closer, her hearing improved, although she never got Carl's last name right, and our relationship seemed to remain a mystery to her.

Once she showed me some pillows she was sewing for her relatives. They were mostly out of modest patchwork, except for one that was made of electric pink satin with big flouncy ruffles. "Hit's for Lester Rhodes, Myrtle's boy in Sneads Ferry." She rolled her eyes in exasperation. "He's a sissy."

"Well, it's real pretty," I said. "He'll like it fine."

She just snorted. But deep down in her old bones, she knew about people who are judged disposable by society.

When her newly respectable relations complained about the company she had found herself—Carl and me and the Hell's Angel—suddenly she couldn't hear too well. And most every month, a rumpled little package would appear on our back steps. A chunk of her welfare cheese.

There have been other offerings on the back steps, too. A sack of tomatoes in August, a beautiful mess of greens in November, a bunch of new onions in the spring. These come from John across the street, who lives with Louise in the house with the sign out in front that reads QUIET ZONE SICKNESS. Back when we moved to Vale Street, terrible arguments would come blasting past that QUIET sign, and doors would slam and things crash against the walls. Then a cop car would drive up, or sometimes an ambulance.

Louise and John know of despair, of aching grief, craziness, flight, and loneliness. When John came over in tears and we struggled to figure things out, sometimes I saw in his face my own sorrow; and in their strife, he and Louise, I recognized the pain and confusion Carl and I knew so well.

Today, life in the shadow of the QUIET ZONE sign is more peaceful. John says it's because we listened to his troubles and encouraged him to find his way past violence. But I'm inclined to credit it to the risks each of us has taken to share and trust.

Mostly, our time together has not been so trying as all that. John and Louise often regaled us with tales of their scramble to survive in white Durham. John would grin and bob and shuffle like he had to do when he used to dodge the golf balls out at Hillandale, where he tended the grass before desegregation. Louise told us about her brief career as a maid at Duke, which ended in a flash of insight—"What the hell is I wearing this apron for?!" A question we might all ask ourselves.

John and Louise have both done their time, so when they learned that Carl had something of a record himself, albeit for political protest, our stock rose. And when we got arrested for stealing scrap plywood recently from a condo construction site, they greeted us as if we had once shared their cells in Central Prison. For sure, they knew we were gay, since Carl passed on stacks of *Front Page* and *Gay Community News* for them to start the woodstove with. And their knowledge that in our way we were outlaws, too, kindled a warmth far more lasting than a scrapwood fire on a chilly morning.

Last November, Carl and I stapled plastic over Mrs. Hartel's windows for insulation. Her brother, Iva Lee, was failing from uremia and had come to spend his last days at her place. In December, Carl was diagnosed with AIDS. On January the twenty-first, I stood at his bedroom window and saw the funeral home van parked down at Mrs. Hartel's. The next day, Carl decided to go ahead and take the pills we had collected for him to die.

A couple of days later, I rang Mrs. Hartel's doorbell. After a while, she hobbled to the door and stared out at me from the dark inside. "Well, I reckon we've both lost our brothers," I said. And then with my arm around her stooped shoulders, we walked to the parlor and sat in heavy old rocking chairs by the gas-heat stove.

She had seen the obituary in the Durham *Morning Herald*. CARL WITTMAN, COMMUNITY LEADER, the headline read, and it went on to tell of his organizing work, his writing, and his gay politicking. "I figgered he was that way," she croaked, reluctant to give word to what she had known all along. "But he always was good to me."

After a while, Mrs. Lanier bustled in from across the street. The weatherman had mentioned the possibility of some snow flurries the next day, or maybe the day after, and she was asking to borrow a cup of sugar to make snow cream. Mrs. Hartel and I smiled at each other quietly. Mostly what she needed was to talk about Carl. "He did a awful lot for East Durham," she began.

"And he wrote all them books," said Mrs. Hartel, matching her. The newspaper account was garbled, of course, and our old neighbors brought their own special confusion to the retelling. "President of the Civitans!" Mrs. Lanier escalated. There had been mention of Carl's opposition to the civic center scheme.

Mrs. Hartel rocked forward and spat into her Luzianne can. Then she exclaimed, "Leader of the gays!" Stunned silent, all I could think was, *Well, Carl, we've made it. We're home.*

A few days later John Thomas Satterfield came over, a little drunk. Geoff brewed him up a cup of coffee and the four of us—Geoff, John, David, and I—sat in the kitchen and talked.

At first, it seemed like John and Louise were in trouble again, like old times. But then the true purpose for John's visit became clear.

John has a way of declaiming in phrases, like poetry, which he repeats and varies. And in his way he proceeded to eulogize Carl.

Carl was out in the garden pulling weeds. John had walked through the gap in the back hedge, on his way home from the Peter Pan Market, and he and Carl got to talking. "He talk to you like a man. Just straighten up from pulling them weeds and talk to me like a man."

"He spec me and I spec him. Nobody like that Carl. He was a *good* man. That Carl sure was a good man."

As John's inflections and cadences changed like an old blues riff on that gray January afternoon, I could see the two of them standing in the golden evening light, out in the garden. Carl with his arms and his feet crossed, like he would do, with his head tilted. John holding his bag of groceries in one arm and adjusting his baseball cap, over and over, with the other.

"Ain't nobody like that Carl," he repeated. "He was a man!" I put my head down on the kitchen table and wept. "That Carl was a man!"

Since then, I've had to wear my pallbearer suit again. (I finally went and bought one last year, for the duration.) Mrs. Hartel, who always said she wanted to die out hoeing her garden, ended up in Intensive Care at Durham County General, lashed down like a wild animal, thrashing to pull off the oxygen mask.

I sat between Robert, the saw-sharpener, and Calvin Holsclaw on the front pew at Hudson's funeral chapel. The wobbly soprano sang "How Great Thou Art." I thought that Mrs. Hartel would be pleased how her "traveling clothes" looked in her coffin. That's what she wrote: "My Traveling Clothes" on the Piggly Wiggly bag where she stored the shiny blue dress she had made for herself. A rat had got in and chewed a hole in the skirt. Mrs. Hartel just shrugged and told us to put flowers over it. It looked fine.

Now it's June the twenty-eighth—Lesbian and Gay Pride Day in Durham. Many of you, and Carl, and I have worked hard over the years to create institutions of a culture that we can call our very own. But our community depends on the state of each individual's humanity. Today I thank Mrs. Hartel, John Thomas Satterfield, and Louise Petty for joining hands and hearts with us on Vale Street. From them we have learned much about strength and humor and self-respect in the face of great odds.

I'm sorry I can't be with you on Pride Day to carry a poster, or speak. Instead, I will remember a wrinkled obituary that hangs in a broken frame in the front hall where two old black people live, in East Durham. And in that I will find great pride.

The Epidemic:
A San Francisco Diary

LAURENCE TATE

Were it possible to represent those times exactly to
those that did not see them, and give the reader due
ideas of the horror that everywhere presented itself,
it must make just impressions up on their minds
and fill them with surprise.

—DANIEL DEFOE
Journal of the Plague Year

1.

San Francisco. Fall 1986. The epidemic has lasted more than
five years; most likely it is just beginning. Cases in the city (not
including the surrounding counties) are approaching twenty-
five hundred, deaths almost fifteen hundred. You pick up the
Bay Area Reporter every week and turn to the obituaries. Often
you know the face.

Among scientists, optimists expect a breakthrough in five
years; the consensus is ten. Pessimists, I guess, aren't polled.

Until the past year, I hadn't been much affected. The media, of
course, plus occasional reports about former acquaintances; nobody close. In various ways and for various reasons, I kept a
distance I'd been keeping for a long time.

Among other things, now, I volunteer at the AIDS Foundation.

* * *

On the AIDS hotline.
Man's voice, out of breath. Look, this sounds crazy, but . . .
If a guy . . . came . . . on some food. "Say a cantaloupe."
And if he put the cantaloupe in the icebox. For "around
twenty-four hours." And if *another* guy came along and took
the cantaloupe out and . . . ate it. "Is that dangerous?"

Last Saturday, Ken and I stopped by Terry's grave, on the
way back from Devil's Slide. I hadn't realized it had been so
long—ten years next April.

It's hard to remember a time when healthy gay men killed
themselves.

Terry was thirty-five, in the best shape of his life. After years
of deprivation, he'd had tricks to burn.

Terry was the first, for me; an early warning. I was thirty
then.

Hotline.
"Last week I had sex with this guy and he was kind of, you
know, coughing and sneezing, and, uh, a couple of days later I
started coughing and sneezing too and, uh . . . Do you think I
have AIDS?"

Three or four times, I've seen Doug on the street. (We don't
speak, of course, or acknowledge each other.) He looks thinner
now, almost haggard. I can only speculate: Nobody I know
knows him anymore.

It isn't that I still have any feeling for him; maybe it's part of
middle age. Terry used to hang out with Doug and me. Doug
would cook chicken or spaghetti or we'd go out for pizza or

54

whatever. Sip wine on the back porch in the evenings. The odd picnic in the park. The sort of thing you can't trust your memories of. Nobody was ever that happy, as subsequent events were to demonstrate.

Hotline.

"I'm conducting an estate sale. And I don't know, but I suspect the man may have died of AIDS. What I need to find out is, what precautions should I take?"

(Gas masks, lady. Rubber gloves. Tongs. DDT.)

It's been six months since Jill died. Brain tumor. Very sudden, at forty-two.

Julian called after midnight, from Santa Barbara.

The last three days she was in a "semicoma"; the doctor said she could probably hear us.

We sat by the bed in shifts. I got midnight to dawn.

I tried to sing the lullaby Mother used to sing us. I got part of a verse, and the chorus, but not the rest. Over and over.

"Jilly," I told her, "I don't know what's left. I don't know what I'm doing. You know, I'm sitting here, and the whole world just gets so thin, so . . . like it's just fading. Disappearing. And we're out in space together, looking down. And there's nothing to hold me but you."

Sometimes these days, I think that; sometimes I think that dying is the only weight in the world, the only substance.

After she died, I lay in the spare room till morning with my Walkman, listening to hymns. Will the circle be unbroken. I am a poor wayfaring stranger. Farther along.

My cousin writes from Houston:

"After a week of bursting into tears for no reason and wishing I was still in therapy, I've decided to cut back drastically on work I'm doing with the AIDS Foundation. I used not to believe in burnout (and I still have reservations) but I'm just so *tired* of death and dying."

Hotline.
A man who starts by asking if he's at risk because his lover with AIDS keeps bleeding on the salads he's tossing. (For some reason he's had to have facial surgery; most of his jaw is gone.) The caller says he's on leave from his job as a surgical aide. "I washed the instruments," he says. "Every day my hands were covered in blood." Of the six men he worked with, five have died. His savings are running out; he has enough left to go back East, start over (he's antibody-negative). If he waits for his lover to die, the money will be gone. If he leaves, the lover says he will kill himself.

Yesterday I went to see Noah. He was better, using a walker to go up and down the corridor. Soon he may be able to use a cane, and go home. He says Matthew spends every evening with him. During the day, he sleeps and watches TV. He hasn't been shaved in a while, and has a wild scruffy look. Very unlike him; he doesn't seem at all vain, anymore.
A ward of young men.

Hotline.
From Red Bluff. He's gay, sounds very young. He's been losing weight, having trouble breathing. Diarrhea, night sweats. There are purple spots all over his body. He's getting too weak to work. He doesn't have a doctor.

Cutting my hair, Robbie tells me about a former customer he visited at Davies, near the end. Twenty-eight years old. About the boy's father, really, who'd said, "I don't care what it costs. I'll spend every penny I have. We'll beat this thing." Now, Robbie says, the father sits and drinks. "The mother seems to be handling it better."

It's a form of sentimentality to think that death confers meaning. The pedestrian is run down in the crosswalk, the parachute doesn't open, the growth is malignant, the body is discovered by the cleaning lady. On and on. Contributions may be sent to the designated charity.

It all resists interpretation.

But there's a charge, of sorts, in impending death. (Like the disease-of-the-week TV shows. Athletes dying young, etc.)

That's a factor in all this. Of course.

Morbid curiosity, cheap emotion. Interesting times.

Hotline.

A fifteen-year-old girl, in Sacramento. Her brother is coming home from Reno to die. Nobody wants him to, except her. She says, "I want to do everything for him."

Dr. Sunderland's receptionist is a muscular young man in designer jeans and a gray T-shirt. He smiles and takes my credit card and schedules an appointment for Friday morning. The X rays have been inconclusive; I must wait for the results of the biopsy.

It was, I thought, just a freckle on the inside of my arm. But it slowly got bigger, purplish.

I leave the office and drive to the beach. It's a cold sunny day; surfers in wet suits, joggers, chill wind. I take off my shoes and socks and sit on the sand. Dig my toes into it, lie back.

Mother died last October, in Phoenix. Liver cancer.

After the funeral, the house was full of relatives. I walked out and drove to the grave, paced beside it in my gray suit, getting the cuffs muddy, talking out loud. "Whatever you had to go through," I told her, "you didn't have to go through this. So just shut up." And: "Look," I said, "I used to go to the baths all the time, and get fucked in the ass by strangers." So there. Bitch. Almost screaming this. Cold and drizzle. Funeral wreaths on a patch of mud.

Somewhere in there, I started collecting requiems. Brahms, Verdi, Mozart, Fauré, Berlioz, Britten, Bruckner, etc. Quite a variety.

Now the grave has a marker, with a bronze vase for flowers, surrounded by grass.

It's like they say in the pop-psych books: You get to an age, and there's nobody to watch out for you.

Years and years ago, in the locker room at the gym, two guys, gorgeous clones, overheard in a crowd. One said, "I don't know, there's just so much, and it goes so fast." And the other one nodded and said, "And you wake up one day and you're old."

I was never part of that. There were the baths, the fucks, sometimes the sweaty serenity, the easy talk going nowhere, details that stuck in your mind. But never the Life, really. Never boyfriends (after Doug), never the clubs, the drugs, the parties, weekends at the River. It was a glamorous constellation, far away.

I wonder sometimes what Terry would have made of all this. Does it signify?

Unlikely. Still he couldn't, today, have sneaked down to the Travelodge with a stock of Scotch and seconal; his conscience wouldn't have let him.

A lot of guys with AIDS and ARC work on the hotline. Some with lesions, some with canes, some just very drawn and pale. Aaron probably has toxoplasmosis; they're waiting to see if he gets brain lesions. Leo has peripheral neuropathy. Fred has had *pneumocystis* twice.

Aaron makes the rounds of "alternative therapies," hoping, he says, to pick up new meditation techniques. He's skeptical of a lot of these outfits: "They're very big on blame." He's in the hospital this week; some kind of endocrinology study.

Ran into Tony on Castro. He's into "radical faeries" now, and Men's Liberation. Of, he says, "hundreds" of men in his circle, none have AIDS. He suggests this is related to their "holistic" outlook, and the avoidance of various harmful substances.

Peter thinks it's cholesterol. That's why Asians don't get it. "And only the Westernized ones."

To buy his house, Ken persuaded Brian, a friend in Kansas, to go in with him. They have since had a falling out over money—fair shares of repairs and renovations, value of the work Ken has put in, etc. The impasse has lasted for years.

(So he refuses to do more on the house. Walls and staircases are missing; the new shower is boarded up, half-finished.)

The deed, it happens, was mistakenly registered as giving each of them the right of survivorship. Ken is antibody-negative; Brian, he thinks, has lived more dangerously. "Well," Ken says, "it seems like as good a chance as any."

Hotline.

Soft, tired voice. He's a nurse in Richmond; KS for five months, lesions on his face. Last week, his friend Rafael died of *Pneumocystis*. Since May, he'd been blind.

The talk rambles; I make soothing noises, suggest East Bay referrals. It hits me when he says, "Sometimes you think, why go on."

I scramble for the page on crisis calls as I say, "You're thinking about . . . ending it?" and he says yes. ". . . Now?" He says yes. "Have you thought," I ask, "how you'd do it?" He says he has some pills.

I'm very scared; it's only my third week on the phones; I can't remember what to do. I scribble "SUICIDE CALL" on a pad and push it at Chuck.

I babble and repeat questions. In a minute, he thanks me for my time. I say, "Wait, let's talk about this. Please." He hangs up.

The biopsy is negative (as, in time, is the antibody test). I'll live.

"The whole earth," Eliot said, "is our hospital."

2.

Early spring 1987. The panic has escalated. Hotline calls have doubled; the test sites are jammed.

They come to the Foundation from everywhere, the way they go to Beirut or Ethiopia. Camera crews from the BBC, Sweden, Japan. Journalists, photographers, producers, media bums.

Aaron works on the PWA Switchboard, and is now an international star of sorts. At the hotline, we get the spillover, local TV and some out-of-towners, taking pictures, interviewing volunteers.

In four years, there are projected to be around 300,000 cases in this country, ten times the present number. Two million may be infected now. You think of boats drifting toward waterfalls, the last days of a certain idea of civilization.

My friend Ken says, "Start thinking triage.

"Forget Haiti. Forget Africa. Those people can't be educated, can't be treated. They're gone.

"Because, the way it looks now, of the infected people, some number will get hit by trucks or something before they can get sick. So you'll never get a hundred percent. But you'll get close. Services are already starting to crack. Nobody realizes yet. They think a vaccine will come along, or some wonder drug.

"The only reason AIDS isn't the medieval plague is that, in the developed countries, education will work. Not perfectly. I mean, you can't get people to use seat belts, for God's sake. But it won't be everybody."

I repeat some of this to Aaron. He shakes his head and says, "That's something you healthy people will have to worry about."

Aaron is housemother at a flat maintained as temporary AIDS/ARC housing. Sometimes I have dinner there. Three or four guys around the kitchen table, spaghetti and garlic bread, chatting.

One turns out to know my college roommate, who has gotten into the occult. Another is learning Chinese. One is on oxygen, trailing a long clear tube from room to room. They compare doctors, drugs, social workers.

And I get flashes of this spooky detachment: They're all dying. Soon they'll be gone.

I'm eating with ghosts.

It's a sensation you can get anywhere, these days. There's half-serious talk of lost generations, as in the trenches of another age.

On the hotline, callers ask for estate lawyers, or funeral homes, or the Hemlock Society. You look up the numbers and make the referrals.

In a video store, in the Castro. A tall emaciated guy, wild hair, spots on his face, with a cane. The clerk says, "How are you feeling?"

"Oh . . . you know. Life goes on."

Words and phrases overheard, again and again. Diagnosis. Ward 86. KS. AZT.

And canes. Young men with canes.

There are paper cups, dirty ashtrays all over the house, from the gathering after the funeral. Matthew and I go silently from room to room and out onto the deck overlooking the city. Bright sun, no wind.

He eventually says, "I don't know where to start."

We turn and lean on the rail, facing the house. Matthew is executor of Noah's estate, which is to be liquidated and the proceeds donated to the AIDS Foundation.

"He said you could take what you wanted," I say.

We wander back into the living room. He picks up a glass figurine. "Just something small," he says. He stares at the figurine for a long time; tears run down his face. He wipes them away and says, "Is there anything you'd like?"

"No."

"Let it go," he says. "Like *Citizen Kane* and the sled."

He sits on the couch and lights a cigarette. "Do you know how many houses there are, like this? Antiques, china, paintings. Lifetimes of collecting. . . . Still, the market is always there for the good stuff."

He takes a drag and leans all the way back, looking at the ceiling. "The last time they weighed him, he weighed seventy-six pounds. I don't plan to be that brave. I called that place, that . . . society—"

"Uh-huh."

"They send you instructions. It's easy."

"You're not sick."

"Not yet. But come on—the longer you have it, the worse it gets."

"Matthew, they don't know. Really. And this isn't the time to—"

"Oh shut up. Fuck you. You haven't got it. You don't know. You don't know shit." He is crying again. "I mean, I'm glad. Of course, I'm glad. I love you. But shit . . ."

I move closer to him and put my hand on his shoulder.

"Oh, Larry," he says in a while. "I can't even have a drink." (He's been in AA almost a year.)

With Laura on the beach, below Fort Funston. Scattered clouds, a little chilly. Hang gliders overhead, a bit unsettling, like giant birds. One very high up, in the distance.

"They didn't even pay for my lunch," she says. "The Japanese at least did that."

"I warned you," I say. "Everybody hates the BBC."

"I told you, didn't I, the Japanese asked me if I had anal sex."

"Uh-huh."

"They were really rude. I was surprised."

Laura was diagnosed almost a year ago, with PCP. She volunteers at the Foundation, and does a lot of interviews. Several times, camera crews have followed her around. (At the Foundation, these days, somebody is always being followed around. Laura introduces them as "my entourage.")

We pass a couple of dogs splashing in the surf. "I keep getting these infections," she says. "My cunt is all purple. And it itches." We talk about her health a bit; mostly she's felt okay.

"Oh," she says, "I meant to tell you. I got a letter from Jay." (Jay is her brother.)

"Did he see—?"

"He saw Oprah. He doesn't get up early enough for 'Today.' And anyway, he's very embarrassed."

"Sounds like Jay."

"Well, I thought, if he's embarrassed now, he'd better hope the Japanese show never gets here."

We walk to the point, decide to turn back.

"I don't know what I thought Jay would be like," I say. (Laura and I knew each other in high school, lost touch after college. We met again, at Christmas, in the lounge at the Foundation.)

"It's disappointing," she says. "Just in general. And he got really good on the saxophone. Now I don't know if he plays at all."

We look out at the waves, up at the hang gliders. I count eleven of them, swooping back and forth.

"And then there's Sara. And Mother." She chews on a nail. "And me."

Her little sister Sara was killed in a motorcycle accident in 1969; her mother died of cirrhosis a few years later. Her father is in a retirement village in Arkansas and doesn't communicate with anyone.

"Talk about disappointments," she says.

The wrangling over Ken's house is finally settled; Ken pays eighteen thousand dollars for Brian's share. A factor in the negotiations is that Brian has recently had shingles—a sign of a weakened immune system. At one point, Ken asks him whether there's anything else. "Not at present," he says.

Ken tells me, "I could have held out. There was nothing he could have done. But—"

Hotline.
Deep voice. "I have some information for you."
"Uh-huh."
"This has to get to the top."
"The top?"
"Your top people."
"Okay."
"Now write this down."
"Okay."
Three things, as it turns out, heretofore unsuspected, that cause AIDS. The first is saccharine, the second is iodized salt.
"Now the third one," he says, "you might see some problems with."
"Uh-huh."
"The geography and such."
There's a pause. I say, "What is it?"
"Vampire bats."
He gives me his name and phone number, which I don't write down.

A couple of weeks later, a kindred spirit suggests "moondust."

"Moondust?"

"You know," he says, "like—when they came back from the moon. They brought it."

And so on:

A woman whose husband has received an anonymous letter saying he's been exposed.

A man with KS, "more lesions than skin." His doctor has given up.

A sailor in a special ward in a Navy hospital, for antibody-positives. They're being pressured to admit being gay.

A teenage girl who was raped, anally, by two needle users.

A UC student who's just got a positive result. He's an athlete, with a lover. He cries a long time. (During parts of this call, a Swiss photographer is hovering and clicking, two feet away.)

And one in the bus station in Sacramento, calling on the 800 line. He's broke, knows nobody. His name is Glenn. "I've had a hard life," he says. He "travels around," has gone to the baths a lot. He's twenty-eight.

Diarrhea, night sweats, fatigue, fever, weight loss. White stuff on the sides of his tongue.

Through several calls, I try to find a doctor there, a place to stay. (The public hospital is far away, and who knows if they'd admit him.) No luck.

He says he can spend the night in the bus station since he's got a ticket on to Seattle. But "they won't let you sleep."

Sunday evening, the AIDS/ARC flat.

Andy is thirty-six today. Aaron has baked a cake.

Andy is saying, "So I told that bitch from Shanti, well sure I cut my wrists, but I didn't *mean* it. Just seeing the blood, I almost passed out. And there wasn't that much."

"Andy," Aaron says, "we're eating."

"I know that, but I was only making the point that I was a little out of it, at the time, and I think they ought to understand that. I mean, it isn't that *uncommon*." He is having trouble getting into a permanent residence because he is considered unstable. His wrists are still bandaged.

"I am not crazy," he says. "I have a fatal disease. A very frightening fatal disease."

"You poor thing," says Bob. Bob is the one with the tube.

"Oh, hush. It's my party."

Later Andy says, "This place would be so great for a TV series. A comedy. Like "M*A*S*H," with wacky characters all over the place and—oh—say, the board of directors is coming by and somebody's locked in the bathroom with a straight razor and somebody else is shooting up and there's a fistfight in the kitchen and they get all tangled up in their oxygen tubes and . . . that sort of thing. Jim Nabors could be the housemother. And there'd be lots of guest stars because, you know, nobody lasts too long."

Sitting on Aaron's bed, in his room. He is uncharacteristically down.

"Life keeps shrinking," he says. "I'm always so tired and I fight to get up and get out and—oh, somebody dies and it's not even the grief so much as the shrinking. Something else you've fought for, and it's gone. Always closing in, to a bed you can't get out of. Then you're gone, too.

"I'm so scared, Larry. Five years from now, nobody will remember any of us. They'll have problems of their own. And who do we remember, from five years ago? They were dying then."

"I'll be here. I'll remember."

"I guess. But you'll burn out. You have to. Memorial services just don't draw the way they used to. Not for anybody."

On the street, I run into David. He had ARC for years, was recently diagnosed with PCP.

Over the weekend, he says, he had some sort of blackout. "I just lost it," he says, and was found at 3 A.M. by a bartender he knew, wandering on Market Street. "I was sitting on the sidewalk bawling, that's the last thing I remember." His doctor says it was "initial shock" at the diagnosis, not uncommon, and may recur. "He told me to keep a card in my wallet."

Old business.

One afternoon, I catch a glimpse of Doug in the Safeway parking lot; he's got a tan and looks healthier, as if he's been working out.

There's a letter from Julian inviting me to his wedding, in July. (He's marrying one of Jill's doctors.)

And on Sunday in April, around the time of the anniversary, Ken and I take flowers to Terry's grave, which we have a hard time finding again.

Hotline.

His five-year-old son has been molested by a ten-year-old, who in turn was molested by his junkie father. I ask what he means by "molested." He says, "Penetrated anally."

I check with Pat, who says that, even if the ten-year-old produced no semen, there might have been blood exchanged.

*   *   *

A husband and father from Orinda who's gone to adult bookstores for sex. I tell him oral sex is comparatively low risk. He says, "There was the other . . . a couple of times." Active or receptive? ". . . Both."

He hasn't taken the test, is afraid to be seen at a clinic; also, of course, he's afraid to know. "I'll lose my wife," he says, "my kids, my job, my house. The whole thing."

He's twenty-four. The Army has just rejected him because his antibody test was positive. His wife is eight months pregnant. I think maybe there's a mistake—how would he have been exposed to the virus? "All the worst ways," he says.

He asks if he should take out life insurance.

On and on.

Almost summer.

Another round of birthdays, this month. Aaron says, "People are living longer. Two years ago, they told me I had six months."

We're in the PWA office at the Foundation. Laura has stopped by. "They told me to make funeral arrangements," she says, "do the power of attorney, like I barely had time. Any minute, wham, goodbye—you know? Really scared me."

Aaron says, "I guess they mean well. They don't want people winding up unclaimed in the morgue. But all that happens is everybody freaks and runs around doing a lot of crazy denial, right when they need to be getting themselves together."

"I mean, you have to be realistic, sure," Laura says. "Nobody lives forever. But—"

A tall bearded man sticks his head in the door. He is with an Italian camera crew and wants to interview Aaron. (He doesn't realize who Laura is; she says, "Just passing through," jumping up and grabbing her coat.)

As in other international trouble spots, life goes on.

3.

Fall 1987. Coda.

I don't hear from Laura for weeks. Eric (her roommate) says she has a skin infection, blisters all over. Finally she calls. "Well, actually, it's been kind of grim. Oatmeal baths. A lot of the time, I couldn't do anything." Now her skin is healing, but she's tired.

I say I'd like to see her.

"No, sweetheart. I want to hole up. Till I'm better."

A couple of days later, Eric calls from 5A. Laura has some kind of fungus in her lungs. They've put a tube in her chest.

When I get there, she's throwing up in a plastic basin that Eric's holding. She keeps saying, "Jesus, Jesus."

After awhile, she lies back. "Oh Lord. This really is no fun."

Two nights later, a tall balding man follows me into Laura's room. She's sleeping.

"Hello, Larry," the man says. I realize it's Jay.

In the lounge, he says, "The hospital called. She put me down as next of kin. Which is surprising."

An older woman comes in and gets some milk from the refrigerator. "For my son," she says.

Jay says, "My sister is here."

"Oh. The woman in Fourteen."

Jay nods.

Back in the room; Laura's chest hardly moves. Jay says, "I have to find out what to do." I look at him. "About . . . the arrangements. The shipping and everything."

*   *   *

Aaron staggers, sees double, forgets things, loses more weight. He mentions "making some decisions," and has the pills saved up.

Almost winter. I pick up the *Bay Area Reporter* and there's Doug. The write-up mentions a "brief struggle" and lists three friends he "will be missed" by. No lover, apparently.

Hotline.

Walnut Creek. He says, "The son of a guy I work with just died. Of AIDS. I mean, he knew it was coming. We talked about it. And . . . What do I say? What do I do?

"He was my age," he goes on. "Twenty-eight. And . . . I never knew anybody who died before."

I try a few platitudes; he cuts in. "I didn't know who to call. I figured maybe you guys . . ." And repeats, "It's just, I never knew anybody who died."

"I Want to Tell Them:
Do You Love Your Children?
Bring Them Home"

E. J. GRAFF

They're ordinary working people, the kind you'd stand behind in the grocery checkout without paying much attention, ordinary Italian Catholics whose four-room home is filled with prayer cards and statues of Jesus on the cross. But faced with extreme circumstances, John and Josie Politano rose to a quiet heroism. When they learned their son was gay, they made him understand that he was, first and foremost, their son. And when they learned he had AIDS, they nursed him themselves, in their home, until his death.

The Politanos wanted their son's death to mean something. And so they insisted to the *Cape Cod Times* that AIDS be listed in his obituary as the cause of death. After the paper sent a reporter to interview them, the Politanos sent the clippings to *Bay Windows*, a paper their son had read, hoping to reach other families facing the same tragedy.

I met the Politanos in their Falmouth home, less than a month after John, Jr., died on September 25, 1986. John's bedroom was still much as it had been when he was alive. His oil paints and pastels, his half-finished painting of his father, were heaped around the easel; his favorite tapes were piled on his

·dresser; beside the crucifix over his bed was a banner that read
WE LOVE YOU JOHNNY BOY. His hat, his photos, and his guitar
were still in the room; his canaries, Caruso and Angelina, flit-
ted around their cage behind the kitchen table.

They welcomed me into their kitchen, served coffee and tea
and coffee cake. At times crying openly, at times gripping each
others' hands, always without shame or apology, they told me
the story of John Arthur Politano, Jr.'s life—and his death.

"See," Mr. Politano began, "I grew up and seen people that
were gay. It never bothered me; it never offended me in any
way. I mean, I've seen times when people even went after
them, chasing them, giving them a licking. I resented that; I
really hated that. When the Korean War first started, I was up
at the front for fourteen months, and we had a gay guy that
was up at the front with us. Whatever I felt, whatever I seen,
whatever—he felt the same thing. I don't remember anybody
harassing him, bothering him. We never used the word *gay*,
either. He never bothered anybody. He had his own special
life, and we all got along good.

"John was adopted at three months. My sister was his blood
mother. She had a hard time with life. I didn't like the way she
lived—that's her business—but my nieces and nephews, that's
different. She'd come home drunk and beat them up, and so
on. One day my [other] sister went up there and found John
with all the other kids, being pretty well mistreated, and she
went up there and got all the kids."

Mrs. Politano explains that the sister called and said she
couldn't take all seven kids in. "I said, 'Wait, I'll be right there,'
and I hopped on the bus and went over, and I took Johnny."

"When Johnny was eleven," Mr. Politano went on, "next
door to us we had this gay couple that moved in. They were
seniors. They were all right. But I, I heard so many stories that
they go after little boys, and Johnny was eleven. And I called
them a name—not to them, but I said it in the house—'I don't
want those people bothering my kid'—I don't even like to use
the name, but it was 'queer.' I said, 'If they look like they're

near the kid, you let me know.' And that's the first time I ever struck out against the gays.

"I got corrected a long time ago about that. After I found out that Johnny was gay, him and I sat down and we did a lot of talking. I says, 'Johnny, what's this about the gays? Do they go after little boys?' He says, 'Dad, the ones that are heterosexuals that go after little girls have a problem.' He says, 'We have some gays that have a problem, too. Whatever problems you have with heterosexuals, incest or whatever, you have the same problems in the gay community as well.' He explained a lot of things to me like that."

"We were close, the three of us," Mrs. Politano said. "We could talk about anything and it was family. If he had something to say, he had the right to voice his opinion, too."

"The only things was," Mr. Politano continued, "when Johnny was eleven, he heard me call them queers—and Johnny told me, later, he says, 'I started liking boys, I started liking my teacher, when I was eleven years old.' And I said, 'Do you remember when I said that about them next door?' And he said, 'Yeah, I remembered that, that's why I never said nothing.'"

"That made it even worse for him," Mrs. Politano said.

When John was thirteen, his birth mother told him the story of his birth and adoption. He ran away. After two weeks, he called from New York and returned home. He told the Politanos that the shock of learning he was adopted had driven him away. But he kept running away, over and over, for years.

"One time when Johnny was away and I was really lonesome for him, I sat down on his bed," Mr. Politano said. "That was the closest I could get to my son." Politano had reached down in the mattress and pulled up a gay magazine. "I was very shocked. I trembled all over. I tore that magazine into a thousand pieces and threw it in the barrel and then covered it up with newspaper so my wife wouldn't see it.

"To know that people are gay, that's their business. But to find out your son is gay, you do some heavy thinking. What happened? I bought him some boxing gloves and a punching bag—maybe I came on too strong when he was a young kid, you know? Was that the cause of it? I couldn't figure it out. So I called a priest, I said, 'I think my son is gay.' He wanted to know if I accepted it. I said, 'I don't know, I don't know what it's all about, I got to find out more about this.'

"So I did, I found out. I got some literature. I put it over the airwaves on WBSN in New Bedford's talk show, to get the pros and cons. I heard a lot of people that were against the gays. Then I heard a lot of guys that get on there and that was gay—they give you something to think about.

"But could I approach Johnny and ask him if he was gay? I couldn't do that. I didn't have the courage. For a whole year.

"One day he came home and we sat down to have a game of chess. I didn't even know how to say it. I don't even know if I said it right. But it was something like—'If you're gay, I don't care. If that's why you're running away, well, so what? Big deal.'

"He was so shocked. He jumped up and turned his back to me. I went over and repeated what I had said, and he turned and looked at me. He had tears rolling down his cheeks and we hugged each other. We both cried.

"After that he stopped running."

Mrs. Politano added, "About a year later, he told me that John was gay, and I just said, 'So? He's my son, regardless. He's still my son.' And then John used to talk openly to me about it. If I had any questions, I'd ask him, he'd tell me, or he'd get us literature."

After high school, John, Jr., joined the army and was stationed in Oklahoma. After only a few months, his commanding officer was changed. Upon learning that John was gay, the new officer called Mr. Politano to ask him whether he knew. The officer said he felt it was his duty to inform the parent. "So what?" Mr. Politano answered, telling the officer that the gay man he had served with in Korea had "seen what we seen, he felt what we felt." Nonetheless, John was forced out of the service.

John, Jr., spent time traveling around the country, settling for awhile in San Francisco, where he met Everett and began a relationship that lasted several years.

"He explained to me," Mr. Politano said, "it's more than sex, it's love, just like with the heterosexuals. You want to touch him because you love him. You want to have sex with him because you love him."

John and Everett were having a hard time making it financially in San Francisco. The Politanos invited the couple to come live with them in Falmouth. John and Everett moved into the Falmouth house in October 1984. A year later, John went into the hospital for a week with pneumonia.

Mrs. Politano said, "I went in there to see him, and he told me he had something to tell me he did not want me to tell his father. I said, 'What's the matter, John?' He said to me, 'Mumma, I have AIDS.'" Despairing, Mrs. Politano pleaded with her son that she could not possibly live with that news without telling her husband. But John insisted, arguing that he didn't want to endanger his father, who has a debilitating heart condition.

Mrs. Politano kept the secret for a week. But when Mr. Politano, concerned by her morose and silent behavior, demanded to be told what was wrong, she told him.

"I got so angry I punched the cross and I broke it," Mr. Politano said. "I was angry, because Johnny was our only son. And it had to be him." He told his son that he knew. "Johnny was crying and yelling at the same time. 'Why me? Why me? Why did it have to be me?' Him and I were just hugging and crying, you know, and my wife ran over and was hugging the both of us, the three of us were crying."

Mr. Politano had first begun paying attention to AIDS after Rock Hudson died. "That movie actor, Rock Hudson—I really felt it then. I liked him. That was when I started paying more closer attention to what was in the papers and what I heard over the news, and started telling John to get a physical and make sure everything was all right."

Not long after that, his son had told him of meeting someone with AIDS. "Johnny was telling me that when he was in New

York before he even knew he had AIDS, that he was at this party, and there was this old-timer there who had AIDS, a very rich man, and he was buying everybody drinks, everything was on the house. And everybody knew he was dying of this disease called AIDS. And Johnny felt so bad for this guy, he went over and gave him a good hug, because the other gays just kind of shied away from him. When Johnny found out he had the AIDS, he was devastated, because he remembered that old-timer."

John was the first AIDS patient that Falmouth Hospital had. "The nurses treated him like a king," Mrs. Politano said, "bringing him videos, newspapers, sitting up with him when he was upset. The medical staff researched AIDS intensively in order to provide him with the best possible treatment."

John recovered from that bout of pneumonia but had to return to the hospital in November. During that time, the friction between Everett and the Politanos mounted. The parents felt that Everett was mistreating their son. "He was cheating on him, and that wasn't right," Mrs. Politano said simply.

When John was released, Everett talked him into moving to Dorchester, where John could be treated at the Deaconess Hospital. While living there, John was assigned an AIDS Action Committee (AAC) worker. But there was trouble between Everett and John. Mrs. Politano feels that perhaps Everett couldn't face living with someone with AIDS. In May 1986, John called his parents and asked to go home.

"I was taking him back and forth to the Deaconess Hospital in Boston," Mr. Politano said. "His doctor told me he had less than a year to live—about five months according to the symptoms, problems with his kidneys.

"He came to the point where he was too weak to go [to Boston to the Deaconess] any longer. 'Mumma and Dad,' he says, 'I want to be home when I die.' And we told him. 'You got it.'

"That's when we had Hospice. The Hospice nurse that we had, her name was Verna, and if it wasn't for Verna, well, I just don't know. If it wasn't for Hospice to tell us what was happening and what was going to happen, to prepare us for Johnny's death—well, it was hard, believe me, knowing that no matter what Mother and I did, that he was going to die anyway. We let him know that even though we knew he was going to die, and he did, that we were there for him, and we'd do the best we can."

The Politanos got all the information on AIDS they could from the AAC, especially relying on the book *Living with AIDS*. The Hospice workers taught the parents, particularly Mrs. Politano, how to care for their son physically. Hospice also helped in many concrete ways, such as bringing new sheets and arranging for the donation of a new washing machine when the Politanos' broke down. Not everyone in Falmouth was welcoming. Word leaked out that John had AIDS. "We were getting harassing phone calls and everything," Mr. Politano said.

Mrs. Politano went on, "We don't know who they were, they never gave names. They'd just call up and say, 'We know your son has AIDS, get him out of town before he contaminates the whole town.'"

"They were mostly women," Mr. Politano said. "I'd just hang up. It didn't bother me really. What bothered me was— what if John picked up the phone?"

Early in the summer, Everett left for California, telling John he was going for only two weeks. But Mrs. Politano said, "Johnny knew he was gone. He said to me, 'Mumma, you've got Daddy, Daddy's got you—but I don't have anybody.' He used to ask me if somebody that had AIDS, if he had no place to go, could he come here? And I said, 'Sure. I'll take care of him.' And we would. I don't know if we would do it now, but if it would have helped Johnny, I would have done it, if he had found somebody."

The extended family of sisters and cousins and grandparents had accepted John when they learned he was gay. But they dropped out of sight when they learned he had AIDS. "In August we had a birthday party for John," Mr. Politano said. John was turning twenty-four. "We invited one hundred and twenty people. It was a kind of goodbye party for Johnny. Maybe twenty-five, twenty-six people came."

"And none of the family!" Mrs. Politano said emphatically.

Mr. Politano continued, "Johnny's gay friends came, and some of his old friends from school, and some of our friends. But not one of the family came to the party." John asked his parents to try to forgive the family for his sake.

The Politanos showed me pictures of John before AIDS struck. The pictures show an impressively built, good-looking young man, confidently wielding a pool cue or posing on a New York bridge. They showed me also the videotape of him made by his AAC worker, Suzanne, in early August, and pictures of John at the birthday party. There I saw a shockingly different man, as wasted as a concentration camp inmate—but still functioning. Though thin, though embarrassed that his teeth had been removed when they had begun to rot, he was still able to walk and talk, sing and play his guitar.

But by September, John was able to do little for himself. "I was the one that took care of him," Mrs. Politano said, with Mr. Politano helping her lift and turn John when necessary. "I had to give him his medication, and feed him, and change him and put diapers on him. I'd never let him stay wet. I didn't care if I had to change ten sets of sheets a day. He said, 'Mumma, you look so tired.' And I said, 'Honey, it's no problem.' " When John became too weak to drink, the couple would take turns sucking a little liquid into a straw and dropping it into their son's mouth.

One Monday morning in late September, Mrs. Politano said, "He woke up and he wasn't feeling good. He was all congested. I put the vaporizer on, and I called the Hospice nurse, and she told me to pound his chest and his back and to get as much phlegm out of him as I possibly could. He was too weak; he couldn't get it out. So I put gloves on and was actually pulling it right out of his mouth and his throat. I did things I didn't think was possible that I could do, but I did it.

"The nurse came. She took me into the other room, and she

said, 'He's preparing himself for death, but he won't let go until you and your husband tell him it's okay.' I got very angry. I yelled at her, 'I'm not going to tell my son it's okay to die!' She took both my hands in hers, and she said, 'I'm not telling you to tell him now, but when the time comes, you'll know, and you'll be able to tell him.'

"On Thursday morning, about two thirty, he called me, and he said he wasn't feeling good, he wanted his pills. So I gave him his morphine, and my husband and I sat with him for a while. And then he started not being able to get his breath again, with the phlegm and everything. Meanwhile he had wet himself, so my husband and I were changing him. The sheet ripped, and John fell onto the bed. And we had to pull him up, and we told him we were so sorry, we didn't mean to hurt him—he was so frail that just touching him anywhere hurt him!" Mrs. Politano began to cry.

"We were pounding his chest, and he said, 'Mumma, Daddy, please—let nature take its course.'

"His pulse was racing really fast, so my husband stayed with him and I went out and I called the nurse. The nurse told me to give him a Valium, so I went back in, and he took it. My husband walked out, and I said, 'Johnny, you're so tired, hon, it's okay—Daddy and I will do fine."

Mrs. Politano left the room and then went back in to see whether his pulse had slowed. "I grabbed his hand, and he put his head down and took one breath, and he was gone.

"I said to Dad, I said, 'I told John it was okay'—and he looked at me and said, 'So did I.'

"I guess I got hysterical. I kept screaming, 'I want him back.' I didn't think I'd have the guts to say it. And I just didn't think it was going to happen so quick, I really didn't."

After their son's death, Mr. Politano called the *Cape Cod Times* and insisted that they print "that he died of AIDS. I said, 'I don't want this baloney that he died of a long illness or something.' I wanted them to know why my kid died. He died of AIDS."

Mrs. Politano added, "Because it may help somebody."

That article has brought them over a dozen letters of support and thanks and a request to be interviewed on cable TV. One woman, whose son had AIDS and lived in California, wrote and said that she and her husband called their son and that "they're hoping and praying that he will come home so they can take care of him like we did our Johnny." They told me they hoped that their story might appear all around the country. They want gay people to show it to their families. They want parents to know it can be done.

"I want to tell them: Do you love your children? Bring them home! You won't catch it. Hug them and kiss them and tell them you love them. That's what they need. They need the love and understanding and the support. You don't have to worry. They can eat out of your dishes, if you wash them with soap and water. He used to use my bathroom—I'd just clean it with bleach and water; I never worried. If there was vomit, I'd just pull on my rubber gloves and clean it with bleach and water. The only way you'll get it is if you use the same needle or have sexual intercourse. Love them and make them know it."

John Politano, Jr., was buried in the Veterans Administration National Cemetery in Bourne, Massachusetts, in a casket draped with an American flag. His relatives came to his funeral. "But what good is it after he's dead?" Mrs. Politano asked.

The Politanos remain close to some of John's friends, including Keith and Don, a gay couple who have visited them every weekend since their son's death. The house is filled with mementos of their son: his paintings, his music, photographs, letters of condolence from congressmen Gerry Studds and Bob Nickerson, whose offices had stayed in touch with John during his illness, a certificate sent by Governor Dukakis to honor the "one-man art show" that John displayed at his birthday party. The Politanos played tapes of his favorite songs: "That's What Friends Are For" and "I Am What I Am."

"I feel him in every room of this house," Mrs. Politano said. "If I had my whole life to live over again, knowing what I now know, I would have still taken him when he was three months old."

HTLV-3

ROBERT GLÜCK

A small ache harasses my chest—I've wondered for months if it's muscle tension or a virus. Is it my chest or this office that houses so much trouble? I sit on a card chair, cross my legs, and glance at the other men, studiously incurious; I inhale wicked institutional cheer and exhale collective anxiety. I'm taking the HTLV-3 test because my desire to know if I've contracted the AIDS virus is a little stronger than my reluctance. Five to ten percent of the people infected will probably develop AIDS. I usually write in the spirit of disclosure, but I want to clarify feelings and thoughts *before* my medical relationship to the AIDS crisis is established. The Health Center guarantees complete anonymity; even if I decide to make a secret of my lab report, it will alter the way I see myself and, doing that, alter everything. Like other gay men, to be on the safe side I behave as though I'm infectious. An HTLV-3 positive gives that proposition—with some exceptions—medical certitude, while an HLTV-3 negative puts me—with fewer exceptions—in the clear.

I read the endless AIDS coverage in the gay press and articles in mainstream publications. These reports cannot gauge the accumulating sorrow because no language can express so great a feeling; I get an inkling of its scale in the torrent of factual coverage, a deluge of facts, debated and repeated, as though sheer enumeration could save us. I wonder: Will a cough lead to *Pneumocystis*, headache to lesions, a mark on my skin to Kaposi's? My boyfriend speculates that, like a war, the full effects of the trauma won't appear till the disease is "conquered." Sometimes, in the calmest moments, dozing, an image of myself flashes on my mind's screen: I'm sobbing deeper than I ever have, arms in the air, head thrown back theatrically, as it has never been, as I would never allow.

Immediately, I have an impulse to make comparisons and draw morals, to deflect attention from the real trouble, to give a past tense to what can't be fathomed. Anxiety demands a universal to escape itself. All right: AIDS is the disease of the Eighties. Why? Well, the destruction of the immune system is an allegory of the breakdown of "basic structures" now experienced by our country and the West. Or: AIDS is bad news from a remote yet governing part of the body (the immune system, the CIA) and I theorize that the virus was concocted by one of the more feverish outposts of government-sponsored research. Or: AIDS resembles radiation poisoning's silent decomposition, its scientific unwholesomeness and cataclysmic forecast for all people. Or: AIDS is the result of sexual imbalance—we were unnatural or too natural (a death's head leers from the crotch.)

These interpretations are foolish and comforting, as though finding *what exists* were the same as inventing a moral, as though at some moral's bottom line I'd stop being dazed and scattered. I can't supply meaning to a catastrophe whose real life takes place in the microscopic distance (so near it's far) where viruses are normal and *my* existence is an unlikely game of creation and destruction without any stakes. I feel this chemical remoteness to be the void in its mechanical uncaring and its absolute precondition for my existence. Why ask it for comfort when it illustrates the opposite, that is, the improbability of life. I discover this solitude when I lie awake, aware of my existence, wondering if my breath is labored or shallow, if I feel exhausted or just fatigued, wondering if I should associate the operations of my body, the deep hum or tension that is myself, with the workings of the virus.

AIDS must be seen as this rent in the fabric of life, personal and public. Like other catastrophes, AIDS heightens our lives in a way that we would never want. I'm cast into the region of the uncanny, where animate and inanimate blur. I tell myself, I can't die this way, but of course I can. A sense of destiny asserts itself in the face of so many blighted ones—the "me" avid to continue being comes forward.

With that in mind, can I manufacture some historical perspective? During the late sixties, I, and others, glimpsed Utopia for a moment. We saw that the world was the world, not someone's interpretation of it; that life was the fulfillment of itself; that our destinies—our selves—were our own. This revolutionary idea appeared at once on different fronts, and American identity revamped itself. Actually, we merely claimed the happiness and freedom that were promised to us throughout our childhoods in the deceptive fifties. For me, a budding gay man, the new identity meant sexuality. The rules an invisible world made for me had become opaque; I could see they were obviously invented for someone else's benefit at the price of my own emptiness; they seemed to disappear in a burst of laughter. First, we created a mental and geographical terrain in which we could know each other and be known, could recognize gestures and share meaning; second, our sexuality provided a sublime to transcend and dissolve those newfound selves.

In short, it was gay community—well-organized, inventive, imperfect, equipped for the Seventies and Eighties, that is, for urban life, and subject to its pluses and minuses. Unlike older communities, it thrived in an urban setting, in commercial institutions like bars and baths and cafés; it added its own chapter to the history of love in those decades. What other population could respond to urban anonymity by incorporating it into the group's love life as anonymous sex? To the degree that my own aroused body expressed the sublime, it broke every social contract, while the invitation to the sexual act unified a community and was its main source of communication, validating other forms of discourse. A gay cookbook? Put a naked chef on the cover. The task of being the American libido more or less passed from Blacks to gay men. Gay Christmas?—naked Santa. As we created the community, it taught us a new version of who we were, then we became it. This shift in perception about oneself is almost mystical, with the implied reordering of priorities.

Inevitably, a reaction. The new model showed us that the sexuality we had thought *we* discovered was actually a twentieth-century invention, part of an ongoing specialization process—as specialized, in fact, as the twentieth-century version of heterosexuality. Science and authority shape these identities as much as we. Moreover, the sexual revolution peaked and declined well before the onset of AIDS. Finally, identity and consumerism share an equal sign more than ever before— urgent greed, as though the American bandwagon were pulling out for good: yuppies, guppies, an impoverishment of life for which we feel rightly ashamed. Gay community incorporates commodity life into its dynamic, as it did anonymity. Still, where are the selves we discovered, the selves that were discoverers?

It's easy to show that the world is distant, life is distant, we have the vocabulary for that: disjunction and pastiche. (Retro modes inform architecture, fashion, politics—let's get *back* to America. The big movies are wry reworkings of the old genres: *The Shining, Silverado, Star Wars*.) But a touch is itself, a meeting place for the body and the sublime; it disregards language which wants to generalize, negotiate. This unique "meeting place" also describes death (if anything does). That's why observance both of sex and death can function as a community sublime. To make death general, to say ten thousand died of

AIDS, is an example of how language lies. Each death is beyond language.

And yet: Ten thousand have died, more on the way. I imagine—with inescapable racism and also because it's true—epidemics always happening in the Third World. Our last scourge was the Spanish flu in 1918–1919, which killed 500,000—but doesn't the past in this respect resemble a Third World country? Now gays bear the contempt that the USA has for anyone in trouble. Reagan won't associate himself with homosexuality or a disease. It's a public impulse to silence that affects everyone. I'm still a little shocked when I see the word *homosexual* in the papers, let alone AIDS, and how confusing to associate the national libido with death.

"Ten thousand have died"—an example of how language lies in articulation and Reagan lies in silence. In bed, when I listen to my body for distant alarms, I am in a time and class by myself. Still, AIDS creates such magnitude of *loss* that now death is where gay men experience life most keenly as a group. It's where we learn about love, where we discover new values and qualities in ourselves. Death joins, if not replaces, sex as the community sublime. We used to have the baths, now we have the Shanti Project and other volunteer organizations that institutionalize the approach of death, and AIDS support groups, and safe-sex clubs, where sexuality is framed by the AIDS crisis. A sex-slave auction benefit for the Shanti Project certainly deserves it own exegesis under the heading MIX-AND-MATCH—and there's telephone sex, changes in sex practices even between longtime lovers (sex acts also have a history), the innumerable AIDS journals and recountings. I read the obituaries in the gay newspapers instead of the sex ads. Stories about AIDS patients and treatment are passed around, traded, repeated; they help me in my solitude; they are the very matter that creates community, gives it its character, its form and being.

But everything disperses before the question: Will I die

soon? For that reason, it's an unfair question; it breaks the social contract—and it's the only sensible question to ask. What other purpose does the mind have, if not to navigate the body safely through life? Back to the Health Center: a taste of adrenaline thins my saliva. My heart beats; I flip magazine pages; a nurse calls my number; she finds a vein; it fills a test tube. I always feel self-love whenever my blood appears, in a vial or as a taste in my mouth or when it surfaces through a cut or a puncture. These days, my blood is an impressive and dangerous substance. It stands alone now, at attention in its test tube like a Messenger from *The Egyptian Book of the Dead*. It's hard to remain clear when a jackal-headed scientist weighs my heart against a white feather. In two weeks I will learn the results. Five to ten percent—or is it fifteen?—of the people who encounter the HTLV-3 virus will develop AIDS. I hope I can get out of this alive, the mind says, referring to life and not *able* to imagine alternatives.

Liz Taylor, Live!

STEPHEN M. CHAPOT

It's another late L.A. summer's day. An omnipresent sun rakes down Wilshire Boulevard, casting long shadows across the sidewalks. Everyone in the streets has sunglasses sutured to their faces, regardless of their fashion coordinates. I often imagine that were they to remove the glasses, you'd catch a glimpse of two burning hot coals. A couple of joggers in shorts and togs pant by on their way to a bloodfeast. Tonight is yet another fundraiser for AIDS Project/Los Angeles (its "Commitment to Life" show, Part Two, September 20, 1986).

The event has been hyped for months, the ticket price so extravagant it all but eliminates the average person from attending. The absolute trump card of the evening is, of course, Elizabeth Taylor. She's getting another award for her work hawking for AIDS donations. This little lady's been responsible for generating millions of dollars, ostensibly for AIDS research.

If I met her, I'd ask her, "Where's the money, honey?" Maybe tonight I'll get my big chance.

Our destination is the restored and reopened Wiltern Theatre. It's really a building out of time in L.A.'s steel and glass downtown, a green-tiled temple dwarfed by the surrounding office buildings. Walking up the red carpet, past the brilliant lights, I knew those sunglasses would be good for something. Our tickets are waiting conveniently at the will-call window.

88

We're all covered in sweat and stardust. Everyone, even the doorman, glitters.

The theater's lobby is festooned with enough flower arrangements to make even Alexis Carrington wince. The floral designers must think we're eight feet tall—the most beautiful blossoms can only be appreciated by looking down from a teeming balcony. From the height of a wheelchair, it's all wasted.

Long tables covered with piles of hot and cold finger food snake into the lobby's recesses. They're all manned by good-looking Valley boys and girls dressed as French domestics. Everybody is drinking, really putting it down. It's all free champagne.

The room is crowded. The crowd is hot. People kiss in venerated cheek-to-cheek Hollywood fashion, hug and chatter. Posture and gesture are everything for this show, an imitation Oscar night. There are stars and voyeurs assembling.

Some of us haven't paid for our grand entrance, though. We have "gold cards," the distinction being dubious. We've been given passes, gratis, by the AIDS Project. Our role is to hype the organization with the guests and to dress the place with a few well-worn and untanned faces. As I enter, I feel just like a terrorist casing the executive lounge at an airport. I am lost among the stars.

All around me there are actors and personalities, some of them celebrity ushers for the evening. All the stars party together. All it would take is a little bomb hidden in my pocket and I could blow a huge hole in American prime-time TV. All three networks would go dark in a flash. PBS would finally be king of the airwaves. The dead would go into immediate regional syndication, where the real money is, anyway.

Everyone can use that career boost that comes from personal tragedy; it has certainly worked for me. The most exciting thing you'll discover, when you walk up and confront these people, is that they all act exactly as they do on their shows. Here's William Shatner in agony trying to make a point. Tony

Danza's looking tough over by the stairs. Ali McGraw, an actress of no socially redeeming value, stands alone. John Lithgow looks just like the undertaker he was born to play.

For the disabled, TV is the last sanctuary, always bright and clean and colorful, and unchanging. It's small wonder we think we know these people intimately. We do. The trouble is, none of them has ever heard of us.

I've been handed the perfect opening line for this party. "Hello, Mr. So-and-so. Having a good time? I have AIDS." I'm sure they all expect this to happen, and they're pretty casual for the most part. They should be. As professional thespians, they've had a zillion opportunities to manufacture an emotional response.

But who's the star now? I'm the closest many of these people will come to a case of AIDS. Let's savor my performance.

The few of us who do have AIDS all recognize each other, having met one another at various hospitals, medical offices, pharmacies, or therapy groups. Besides, we've got "the look" and can spot each other across a crowded room.

I nod and keep moving. We all seem to have come here alone, are all shuffling this way and that, staring at the penguined crowd. Eventually, though, we draw together, the attraction of wandering magnets inevitable. Finally, I find myself scrunched in a corner with three other guys with AIDS.

Could this be kismet? Hardly. Our greetings are almost predictable: We've all met before. Most of us are drinking, too, one surprisingly on his fourth glass of the bubbly. I no longer drink, but I'm smoking like a chimney, forced to drop the ashes into my pocket.

Our conversations open edgily. We don't want to hear about another person with AIDS who is doing badly—it's always so ominous—but we also don't want to hear that everyone's doing better than we are. Each of us imagines himself as cast as the sole survivor, meaning the rest of the auditions will have to go. We are all poker-faced. As Billy Crystal will say later, "It's better to be looking good than to be feeling good. And, my darlings, you know who you are."

I start.

"Before, I was never quite sure whether I was actually living my life or whether it was all a movie. Now I'm sure' it's all a movie. When I was well, I didn't know anyone who was sick. Now that I'm ill, I don't know anyone who is well. The only topic I know anymore or can talk about is AIDS. I just don't have anything in common with 'normal' people anymore," I say. "I'm afraid I'm losing my social graces."

Kevin, an avid AIDSophile, is next.

"Every time I turn on my TV set or see anything in print, my blood pressure goes up at least fifteen points. I've gotta cancel all my subscriptions and throw out my home entertainment center. Believe me, I don't need any more education. Just look at this bunch. It's all the appearance of a lot of action and concern—but for us it's just a big black hole."

Then Albert.

"Frankenstein. I feel like Frankenstein. They pump me full of these toxic drugs and then tell me to stay to be available for any up-coming experimental programs. Then they deny me the new drugs because of previous drug involvement. Christ, they want AIDS patients who have no signs of the disease for these tests. What are they going to do with the rest of us?

"Now we're all supposed to take the new drug, AZT. I swear, gay restaurants are going to start looking like a rerun of *The Stepford Wives*, little alarms going off and everyone pulling out a bottle of pills. First they ask who's going to pay for this and do you have insurance, then they use you to collect their data and throw you out like an old hypo."

Raul is last.

"I feel like Kate Hepburn, I hate doctors. I don't think I have any more decent blood to give them. I can't tolerate another pointless clinical interview. Doctors, you can't live with them and you can't die without them."

Just then Whoopi Goldberg waddles by, rather bowlegged, saying she has "Liz Taylor up my ass with the rest of my jewels." She starts me wondering: What can you catch from that? Liz, Queen of the ball, is in the wings complaining of a toothache and threatening to pull out of the show. I knew it. It just had to happen. It wouldn't be Hollywood unless some damn dame threw a star fit. The APLA honchos are mortified and she recants.

Our conversation resumes.

"I hate Louise Hay. I swear that woman floats," one of us says. "She's walking around here like some Olympian goddess. Word is that she sold Avon before she realized there was a fortune to be made from us. I hate that Norman Cousins, too. He can go sink in his pleasure craft. I hate all these people who think we needed this disease in our lives to give it some meaning. I say screw all this 'channel your energies crap.'"

We start the standard inquiries about each other's health. Our responses are simple, direct, disturbing.

Albert starts. "I'm okay now. September was a bad month. I've developed parkinsonism from all the drugs that I'm prescribed."

Kevin says he just got out of the hospital, pneumonia again. "It wasn't too bad. Only three weeks."

Raul raises his hand and rolls his fingers into a fist. "I've tried everything: meditation, laying on of hands, healing crystals, having my hair and fingernails analyzed, group therapy— all that positive-thinking stuff—and nothing seems to help. I'm only forced into these weird ideas because medicine has nothing to offer me. I feel lousy, just plain lousy."

Then, we get into our "funniest AIDS story." Kevin is first.

"I know of one guy. He and all his friends were sure that, indeed, he did have AIDS. He went to the doctor and after the usual battery of tests was ushered into the office to hear the results— 'The good news is that it isn't AIDS. It's garden-variety lung cancer. How do you feel about morphine?' The guy just flipped out."

Kevin was another. "I love the one about the aerobics instructor who insisted on leading a heavy workout session after a long day on chemotherapy for his cancer. Five minutes into it, he threw up an entire Mexican brunch on the first two rows of dancing dollies. When they tell you to go home and get in bed after chemo, they're not kidding."

My story concerns a friend in San Francisco who is a legit beauty and fashion consultant. He went down to volunteer as a buddy to AIDS victims and because of his personal demeanor, they keep matching him up with these dying transvestites. You have to be tough to survive these queens—they've found their style and are sticking to it no matter what happens.

He would sit for long hours with these guys with end-stage cancer, who were wearing gold lamé dresses. One would-be ingenue sat flipping through old drag Polaroids and musing, "See these tits. They were *real*. They were *mine*. Now I look like a couple of day-old fallen soufflés."

My friend's biggest fashion challenge came in the form of a twenty-two-year-old Filipino flower who was hospitalized for the last time. This one was a nurse's nightmare: uncooperative, screeching and crying with rage, tearing out his IVs, throwing everything including pee bags out the window onto an unsuspecting public. He'd spit all over the furniture and took to lobbying wads of soiled toilet tissue at the TV set.

Of course, he insisted on wearing a ton of bad makeup and dressing in these filthy Japanese robes. He looked like an emaciated, overpainted Korean Kewpie doll.

The real problem, as my friend saw it, was that this kid had no idea how to do his face. He walked into the kid's room, shooed out the nurses, closed the door, and drew tight the drape.

"I'm going to teach you how to do your makeup," my friend said, hauling out the biggest cosmetics display case he owned. The patient was stunned. His face lit up.

They spent two days in conference, learning how to shade

and contour, highlighting and powdering everything so it wouldn't slide from his face. They dyed his hair, fixed it in a French chignon with two red chopsticks. Someone brought in a diaphanous gown. The difference with this patient was night and day. He died that afternoon, contented, looking like a Polynesian Ava Gardner. Now, that's what I call dignity in death.

My friend is crazed. He went to the Empress drag ball to raise money for AIDS. They had to deliver him on the back of a flatbed truck. He's in the middle of a room crowded with over-the-hill transvestites in shimmy skirts and Monroe wigs, and he's wearing authentic antique widow's weeds with a six-foot-wide hoop skirt.

He says that volunteer work as a buddy does have its rewards. "They all leave me such fabulous clothes in their wills."

Invariably, the talk turns to suicide. We discuss it with an ennui that comes from knowing that the best thing any of us will be remembered for is having died from a pop-culture disease. None of us is surprised at our candor.

"I think I've got it all figured out," says Albert. "I call it twilight sleep. I bought the perfect diameter hose for my auto exhaust. Now all I have to do is find an apartment with a garage. Who wants to die in the street? Does anyone know how to disengage the emission controls?"

Kevin feels differently. "Pills. Pills will do it for me. No muss, no fuss. My doctor is horrified. The problem is that if I get too sick, I'll never get to them and no one will bring them to me. They'll all wring their hands while I go slowly down the drain, but they won't help me get there any faster. Pills are the only way to die on time."

I sigh. "Why not shoot myself at one of these engagements, or maybe I should just light myself on fire and fly down from the balcony like some avenging angel."

Raul finishes his glass in one big gulp. "Just remember to wear clean underwear."

"Yeah," I say. "And don't forget to fast for twenty-four hours before the show." We're all cowards, no one wanting to leave a mess.

As we speak, Madonna rushes by with all of her security oafs and sniffs. "I don't know nobody and nobody knows I'm here." We echo her feelings, having found ourselves strangers in a strange land.

Finally, the chandeliers blink on and off. An icy silence settles. There we are, four very ill men on the edge of a lovefeast.

The show is everything you would expect from this town in a crisis. No one mentions the word *AIDS* until twenty-five minutes into the show, and when it comes, it's mentioned by the director of the AIDS Project. Someone snickers. "She dresses like my old aunt." They present an award to a man in a wheelchair who has brought his own oxygen. This is an audience that gives a man a standing ovation for dying in public.

Suddenly there's a scream from the balcony: "This show is about Liz Taylor? Where's Liz Taylor?" There's nothing worse than a hungry fan.

When Taylor does make her appearance, she promises "to spend the rest of my life fighting AIDS." I chuckle. "So will I, honey, so will I."

This remark elicits stifled laughter from my companions in an otherwise drop-dead-silent house. The show is long. All this standing up and clapping and sitting down—I'm worn out.

I wonder, as it ends, whether I'll see my three companions again. The statistics are against it. They're just nice average guys thrust into an inescapable situation—not unlike so many of today's tired movies. We lose ourselves in the exciting crowd, no more obvious than anyone else—all perfect extras.

As I leave the building, I pray the guy in front of me doesn't turn around. Don't look now. I'm right behind you. I'm the modern-day vampire and I might bite. You want to ship me to an island? Great. Let's take Hawaii.

It's going to get worse for me, for us all. Still, I got my big break. And like all the bad movies haunting the pasts of the stars on parade tonight, I just hope I can live it all down. My only disappointment is that I probably won't be around for next year's big show.

As they say in the business, "This one's got no legs."

I guess you have to earn stardom, living fast and burning bright for the descent. Outside the Wiltern, the Los Angeles air is still, hot, smells familiar. The intersection is just as grimy.

I gotta get out of here. I'm in my role. I gotta go home and bone up. On dying.

Steve

STEVE BEERY

Steve and I tweaked each other's fantasies from the moment we met. It was a case of opposites attracting. He was a big, dark, naturally butch weight lifter, thirty-four and experienced. I was leaner, blond, twenty-two, ready and willing to ride off with some handsome cattle rustler. He told me he'd had his eye on me in the bar for two weekends running, that I reminded him of Parker Stevenson from "The Hardy Boys." He was the reason I'd gone back to that bar; he reminded me of Mike Mentzer from the physique magazines.

Like a lot of musclemen, Steve knew the trick of flexing one of his pecs now and then during conversation—a quick snap inside the tight Polo shirt. I know the pec snap turns a lot of people off. It's corny, and if it's done with so much as a trace of arrogance, it's insufferable. I read Steve's as a wink, a playful call to action, so I snapped back at him and accepted the invitation.

I liked Steve's size and he liked mine. There was a wonderful, exaggerated contrast between our bodies, like a Tom of Finland drawing of a furry Daddy and his smooth-skinned Son. We both like to wrestle and we both liked it when Steve won. We must have gotten together to play a dozen times in that first month. But for all the heat we generated in bed, neither of us felt Cupid's arrow. It wasn't romance.

In the back of my mind an alarm was going off. "Don't waste your time if he isn't lover material," it was saying. I've since discovered that having a lover is gravy. Good friends and a fuck buddy will get you through.

Besides, I lived in town. Steve lived on the Peninsula. He was a jet mechanic with one of the big airlines and he wanted a short commute to his job at SFO. He had three big cars he liked to tear down, and at his town house condominium in South San Francisco he had plenty of room for them.

His politics were as suburban as the rest of him. One night in bed, he told me he felt Jimmy Carter was seriously eroding America's resistance to Communist takeover. I mentally crossed politics off my list of postcoital conversational topics and continued to call him every few weeks for a session of hot, apolitical sex.

Steve was always horny. Half an hour after doing it, he'd have that mischievous look in his eye again. He was already losing the hair on his head; too much testosterone, I imagined. He was a big teddy bear—generous, considerate, unpretentious. He was a Nixon Republican through and through, but when it came to sex, he was democratic.

A typical afternoon get-together would find his bedroom primed for action. He'd have plate-glass mirrors propped against the armchairs, lights clamped to their top edges. Towels would be spread in every direction. There'd be quantities of lube, poppers, ball straps, and cock rings, and fresh packs of film for the Polaroid. Nothing exotic, no dildos or alligator clamps; no doubt our play would seem "too vanilla" to many. Some days he'd wear me out, other times I'd exhaust him; we were pretty evenly matched. I knew other guys who were sexual athletes, but most of them had an air of grim determination. None kept a sense of humor about sex the way Steve did.

There was no fixed pattern. Sometimes we'd see each other twice a week, sometimes not for a month or two. If one of us had a new boyfriend, we always knew when the freshness of passion had worn off; that's when he'd call me or I'd call him and we'd get together for sex and a movie. We saw *Pumping Iron*, to feed my muscle fantasy, and *Blue Lagoon*, to fuel his pederasty.

In many ways, I felt fuck-buddying was an ideal relationship. Since there was no daily routine, there were no hidden resentments, no hurts, no slights, no alienated affection. Gay men, after all, are accustomed to investing different partners and acts with different levels of intimacy and meaning. As far as I was concerned, the fuck buddy was a clear case of instinct triumphing over civilization.

Still, we had our differences. He had his friends and I had mine. He didn't read books and I've never understood what it is that makes a car run. We also differed in our degree of openness about being gay.

Steve wasn't out at work except to a couple of trusted friends. He'd dated women throughout his teens and twenties, and was already entrenched at the airline when, at thirty, he discovered his attraction to willowy blond boys. He thought it advisable to be discreet. I used to tease Steve about coming out, but not too strenuously. After all, his mother knew, and back then I felt that learning to announce yourself, like learning to swim, was something people ought to take at their own pace.

He was only twelve years older than I was, but in some ways he belonged to my parents' generation. He listened to Frank Sinatra and Mantovani records. Though he'd had plenty of experience to the contrary, part of him still believed the old gay stereotypes: that he was the "man," and that his blond boys were somehow the "girls." He found it endlessly funny that a big butch guy like him was gay at all.

It was Steve who taught me about the baths. He'd pick me up after work and we'd check in around six o'clock. We'd start by playing together in his room, to "knock the sweat off it," as he put it. Then we'd explore separately. Later, he'd drive me home and we'd compare notes about who we'd gotten it on with. Since I liked guys who looked like Steve, and he liked guys who looked like me, we could often steer each other toward some good bets.

The baths were ruled by a gentleman's code of conduct that permitted everything except rudeness. Any invitation was declined only with the greatest respect. It was entirely my idea of a retreat—long lazy hours of hide and seek in the corridors, lolling in hot tubs, splashing in showers. The only drawback was the omnipresent thump of the disco tapes.

I learned things my education up to that point hadn't covered: not to mistrust pleasure, nor to read too much meaning into a simple orgasm. All around me, I saw in what infinite variety men's bodies could be good-looking. Sex is knowledge, and even with Steve, who represented an ideal of male beauty to me, I didn't want to be monogamous.

At forty, Steve was manlier than ever. He'd kept up at the gym, and we both agreed that he was on his way to being the world's hottest fifty-year-old. We had each spent time with a couple of different boyfriends, still looking for the lover that never quite materialized. Somehow, through it all, we'd never lost the urge to grab each other's ass.

We fell back into our familiar nonpattern. Steve bought his first VCR and added TV to the mirrors and lights. He'd bring out an armload of porno tapes, full of blond boys, with one or two Colt men tossed in as a nod in my direction. The seductions were my favorite part; by the time the guys on the TV were doing it, we'd be doing it, too. I often found it hard to concentrate on the tapes. Being with him was more fun than watching what those models were doing.

Then Steve met somebody special. Craig was the youngest,

willowiest blond boy he'd met yet. Also, from the way Steve talked, he seemed willing to let Steve's paternal side come out, not just in bed but all the time. Sure enough, Craig moved into his guest bedroom, and with just a twinge of jealousy, I wished them well.

It was the time of the first full impact of the disease they were calling GRID. A year later, Craig got sick. His diagnosis was hard for Steve to accept. He made it clear to the doctors and nurses in the hospital that, where Craig's welfare was concerned, he was the first to be consulted. This was Steve's coming out, and he did it with a fury. He found his identity as a gay man by kicking ass and taking names, trying to save his lover's life.

When Craig died, Steve was devastated. We spent some nonsexual time together—just buddies, helping each other through the night. Every inch a top man, he firmly believed that his blond boys were more at risk than he was. During the year that followed, we hashed out our own version of safe sex. We both liked visual, verbal, tactile play where imagination did a lot of the work. We'd gotten so good at getting each other off, we could, and did, do it over the phone.

Our fuck-buddying was going so well that we decided to risk a week in Hawaii together. Surprisingly, there were no arguments about Republicans or gay rights. I had to give us credit; we'd learned how to coexist peaceably. For a week we thought about nothing but sun, sex, and mahi-mahi.

Steve was pleased when, a few months later, his doctor started testing his T-cell count. "I'm a numbers man," Steve said. "I can understand numbers." It was the mechanic in him talking. When the numbers betrayed him by dropping below acceptable levels, he seemed outwardly unperturbed. He quit work and devoted himself to leisure: his cars, the gym, his new rental unit. He visited his friends in Honolulu for weeks at a time. There, the sun and the sea helped his skin, which was beginning to break out in a splotchy rash; a side effect of low immunity, his doctor said.

After his first bout with *Pneumocystis*, Steve's busy leisure turned into days of television: "Wheel of Fortune," "Black Sheep Squadron," "Inch by Inch." His skin was worse and the anti-itch medication kept him sedated, kept him from feeling horny. From time to time, he'd call and say, "I haven't taken an itch pill today." That meant, hurry on down, get some while it's still working.

I considered moving in with him, to help him around the house. Years earlier, before he'd met Craig, he'd told me a lover was the only roommate he ever planned to have. Now he was talking about taking a roommate to share the house payment. Maybe it was time for us to reverse the roles, time for me to daddy him.

Then I reconsidered. He hadn't liked my seeing him in the hospital. With his friends and family, it was different, but to me he liked to present himself at his sturdy best. I hesitated talking to him about it. We had never been everything to each other; perhaps it was too late now to start. While I was hesitating, his mother gave up her apartment in Redwood City and moved into what used to be Craig's room.

Steve and I are still good, dependable fuck buddies, though for the last couple of months, since his second hospitalization and his problem with his liver, he hasn't felt much like doing it. We've known each other for twelve years; I'm thirty-four, the age Steve was when we met. He hasn't driven his car much lately. When I visit, I take the train to South City and walk up the hill from the station.

In the old days, when he used to drive into town to pick me up, sometimes he'd wear his cross-your-heart leather harness under his jacket, with no shirt, just to tease me during the drive home. One time we were so hot for each other, we didn't even make it to his bedroom. We tore each other's clothes off just inside the front door and fucked in the foyer, in front of his hall mirror.

"Sure wish you were feeling better," I told him last week. "So do I, kid," he answered.

It was the same bedroom I've known for twelve years, but it had changed. Daffodils and get-well cards crowded the nightstand. His inhaler and a dozen bottles of pills filled the old cock-ring drawer. Two bathrobes and a fresh pair of pajamas were laid out, for changing when he has night sweats. I haven't seen the lights and mirrors for about a year. "High Mountain Rangers" was on the TV—Robert Conrad and his blond sons in tight ski pants, the softest porn of all.

I hadn't guessed, all these years, at his real strength. He's thirty pounds lighter, and the contrast between our bodies isn't nearly as exaggerated as it used to be. His biceps have come down, his chest is thinner. I haven't seen him snap his pecs for awhile, but none of his toughness has shrunk. If I want to put him in a fighting mood, I only have to mention Jesse Jackson or some other damned Democrat. Last week, I decided anger would just raise his temperature.

I rode home that night thinking about the positive antibodies my doctor tells me are floating around in my bloodstream. My T-cells, he says, are flourishing. "You're as healthy as a horse," he said a week ago. "Keep doing whatever it is you're doing." I arrived home, and with the satisfaction I used to think only a lover could know, I had sex with Steve in my head, playing old tapes that are still hotter than any video.

The Examination Table

CRAIG ROWLAND

December 1981
Houston

Though no one realized it at the time, I was on the examination table because I had AIDS. As a long, horrible plastic snake was fed down my throat, my anxiety level was mismatched by a lack of physical tension. Heavy doses of Demerol and Valium had smoothed me out.

The department head of Gastroenterology at M. D. Anderson Hospital was treating the esophagitis that had painfully appeared a few days earlier. He explained everything—not to me but to the group of medical students gathered around. I got the top man because my boss, another Anderson doctor, who was to create the AIDS treatment center there a year later, paved the way. They were after a biopsy.

Shortly, we all tuned in to a closed-circuit channel as the high-tech tube with its camera eye lit up a TV monitor on the ceiling. I was watching my first AIDS infection onscreen in living color.

When the procedure was over, my boss, who had been standing by, drove us to a nearby restaurant where our department Christmas party was unfolding. Though I was much too stoned to be there, I floated and laughed through lunch, then went home, returning to work by the end of the week. A simple oral treatment worked in two days and the infection never recurred.

During the following months, I was herded around to other specialists, such as the kind young doctor in Immunology, who told me my immune system was, inexplicably, a mess. He handed me Xeroxes of the first medical journal articles on immune dysfunction among gay men, papers that, as a medical editor at this institution, I had already read with mild interest, then filed away.

These were the old days, when "GRID," as wrongheaded a concept as it was, had just been coined. Everybody was maneuvering in the dark instead of the murky dusk we've broken into today. It was unknown that I was a prototype for this disease.

February 1985
New York

I'd had AIDS for over three years now, however I still didn't know it because my original infection hadn't appeared on the CDC list of AIDS-qualifying conditions.

But I could no longer ignore the small red spot that had appeared on my right forearm a few months earlier. Denial has a thousand faces.

Finally, I pointed it out to a doctor at the New York Blood Center, where my immune system was being monitored monthly for research.

"Yes, I think it's probably KS," he remarked as I looked up from the examination table.

My heart leaped; I flushed. Instantly, all my medical knowledge dissolved. Words, including my own, echoed as if they were coming at me from outer space.

"How can you be sure?" I choked.

"We have to take a biopsy," he replied.

"Do it now," I insisted, pushing at walls, scared I'd lose the courage once I left the office.

"It'll take two weeks; the local labs are all backed up," he explained.

"No, that's torture! I won't have it."

My mind screamed as I staggered home, colors, noises, shapes blurring around me. I leaped up the stairs to my Second Avenue fifth-floor walk-through, and, hands shaking, swore at my inability to line up the key with the lock.

Once I managed it, I jumped on the phone and was lucky to reach Peter Mansell, a doctor, friend, and associate I'd worked with at M. D. Anderson Hospital, ironically, in the Department of Cancer Prevention.

"Peter, they think I have KS, but they can't do a biopsy for two weeks."

He tsked calmly with his characteristic British understatement. "If you can come down here, I'll do it in one day," he offered.

Next Day
Houston

I walked into Peter's clinic office in the hospital and found him hunched over a desk, with his back facing me. He was preparing punch biopsies to torture two of my three little lesions. I offered a weak "Good morning," and its return floated up over the back of his head.

Peter has perfected the sort of manners that require him to open the door for everyone—of both genders. Since we hadn't seen each other for almost a year, I irrationally interpreted his backsided greeting to mean that he couldn't face me because he knew it would be AIDS and didn't want to have to tell me I was going to die, or lie and tell me I wouldn't. Or maybe I'd get a deathly silence. I shuddered and sat on the examination table.

The following morning, he went to the pathology lab himself, rather than wait for a call, and grabbed the report as the ink was drying. Then he phoned me at a friend's apartment where I was staying.

"Can you meet me at my office at ten?" he asked.

"Is it KS?" I squeaked.

"Let's discuss it when you get here."

That was close enough to a yes for me. Grimly, I slumped in the taxi on the way to the medical center.

I entered Peter's offices in the main building, where we had worked together for two years till I moved to New York. Dale, his secretary, greeted me warmly, but I would have none of that, nodded, and silently went to the execution chair in front of Peter's desk, where I waited alone for an interminable five minutes.

Finally, he brisked in from the hospital across the street wearing his white lab coat. I looked up weakly.

"How are you?" he asked.

"You tell me."

He read quietly from the pathology report. "Spindle cell proliferation consistent with early Kaposi's sarcoma," he said evenly.

All my medical knowledge disappeared again as I lurched for the protection of denial like a half-drowned passenger from the *Titanic* holding on to the elusive safety of a broken lifeboat. Even then, after hearing that headline read to me off the front page of the early edition, I kept thinking, Stop the presses!

"Is it or isn't it?" I asked, hoping for a different answer.

"It's early KS," he said.

I was a dead man. I didn't hear anything else he said—something about chemotherapy.

Now, it *was* official. I had AIDS. On the plane back to New York that afternoon, I felt like E.T.

April 1985
New York

The head of Radiation Therapy at Memorial Sloan-Kettering Cancer Center pointed silently and grimly at the examination table, directing me onto it, while talking to an assistant about my ankles, which were being considered for minimal radiation to paralyze a few small KS lesions. My interests in this treatment were mostly cosmetic.

While drawing red lines on my legs, she rattled off specialist jargon at her sidekick, always referring to "the leg," never to me, never looking at me. I wasn't even attached to "the leg," it seemed. I wasn't even there.

"Will there be any side effects?" I inquired as she continued to make a road map on my right leg.

"No," she clipped abruptly.

I asked whether she could do the last lesion on my forearm, too.

"We're just chasing," she said, annoyed. ("Chasing" is when they hunt down a few lesions and zap them; then when more appear, they zap those too, till there are too many and you switch to chemotherapy or something else.)

"Pretty soon you'll get too many to bother with, anyway," she added, flicking salt on the fresh wound.

A week later, two toenails fell off (they grew back) and I could barely walk because of pain on the soles of my feet caused by the radiation. When I complained, she shrugged and walked away. By choice, I never saw her again. Though I had worked at this institution too, this time it did me no good at all.

Almost four years later, I still don't have "too many lesions to bother with."

Even today, I seethe when I think of the bitch.

June 1985
New York

"Purple is your color," said the enthusiastic homeopath as he fidgeted with an ancient contraption teetering on a stand a few feet in front of me.

I like purple, so I urged him on while making inquiries. "What's this all about?" I asked.

"This is one of only a few devices like it that were saved when the government confiscated the rest," he explained. "They threw the doctor who invented it in jail." The precarious condition of the machine was partly explained by the fact that this happened half a century earlier.

"Why did they shut him down?"

"They said he claimed he could cure cancer with it. I find it seems to help with the immune system," he said encouragingly.

A sound like a lawn mower with a valve problem filled the room when he started the engine. He lowered the window shade to cut out the natural light, then carefully rearranged the gels in front of the bulb in the cancer machine till he got the color he was searching for.

"You won't feel anything," he advised as he aimed the light at my chest. "But later, you might have more energy than usual." He left the room for ten minutes while the converted lawn mower bathed me with its eerie purple light.

As I sat in the pleasant glow, I worried that naïve foolishness might have brought me there. How could I judge? By then, the

AIDS business was boiling with opportunity for all kinds of oddballs offering fantastic interventions. I had no idea how to measure the effectiveness of this light, but, then, that was true of almost any treatment.

Since mainstream doctors had nothing but dark predictions to offer, it was heartening and refreshing to deal with a man—charlatan or not—who offered hope. Hope, in fact, had become such a rare item these days, I was game to take it where I could get it.

14 November 1988
New York

Sitting in the pastel waiting room before my first appointment with this doctor, I fill out the standard registration forms—insurance information, demographics, allergies, medical complaints—then turn in the clipboard. I review the three sheets I typed the night before—one listing blood-test results for the past two years, another a rundown of all my AIDS-related conditions, dates, and treatments, the third, questions and comments for the doctor.

Satisfied that papers are in order, I flip open a copy of *Vanity Fair* and stare emptily at a Calvin Klein ad. My mind is far from the melodramatically posed, shirtless guy in the picture as I drift in thought, reflecting on my seven years in the business of staying alive that led me here today.

By now, I think I'm a qualified veteran of this war, with a clear mind about my intentions for this appointment. There are no fires to put out today; I'm here for logistical reasons, to build bridges.

The running dialogue with my doctor of the three previous years has more or less run its course. Instincts urge me to expand resources. Instincts, in fact, have become my most reliable weapon against this disease. Backed, of course, by the medical knowledge I acquired working in two medical centers, the information I gather as a journalist and patient covering the AIDS waterfront, and from the work I did as a founding officer of the AIDS Foundation Houston—knowledge that no longer disappears under pressure.

Because of lack of time, because of the politics of medicine, because of a lack of cooperation and communication within and between medical facilities and among medical professionals, because prestigious journals demand that researchers withhold new knowledge until publication date, because of egos, because of other human factors, I'm more likely to succumb to confusion and red tape than to the disease—unless I develop a strategy for survival.

I learned long ago not to rely on one doctor, regardless of level of trust or expertise. Most of the good physicians are drowning in patients and barely have time just to monitor all of them.

The explosive irony is that in the face of a nightmare that breathes death, contradiction, and ambiguity at every juncture, I've developed a philosophy of living that will have to help me ride out this epidemic.

The days of stumbling blindly through medical procedures under the thumbs of such mechanics as the Sloan-Kettering road-map designer are over. I have definite ideas about patient-doctor roles. I insist on being attached to my body parts.

Since I don't subscribe to a traditional God, or organized religion, or Louise Hay, I am not interested in relying on bibles of any kind. Instead, I've learned to believe in my own judgment and the importance of making my own choices, while trying to realistically organize support systems around me.

I'm jaded and worn and impatient and angry about my disease. I don't care to "learn to love the virus," as some of the alternative types insist, or make peace with it. This is war and somebody's going to win.

In the past, by pressing against the impenetrable walls of AIDS issues that are out of reach—by trying to do it all—I squandered energy, increased stress and frustration, and lost time I could have used more happily. Instead, now I try to identify what's in my control and concentrate on those angles.

In the absence of knowledge and effective treatments, both of which will come in time, I count on this strategy as my line of defense. It's what works for me. I hope this new doctor will accept that.

It must be a real partnership, where my vote is considered as important as any specialist's. Friends say this man fits the bill. . . .

A med tech calls my name, yanking me from my trance. He ushers me to one of those inevitable, fluorescently lighted, stainless, airless examination rooms.

He opens the door and there it is, my newest examination table. I survey it: It's fancy, doubling as a chair with a reclining back. Tan and new-looking, it sits in the very center of an otherwise empty room, like a pilot's seat, a control center. Yet I choose to lean on a shelf as the med tech and I talk.

He opens my empty, virgin file.

"I have to put something on this page," he says politely, while displaying a blank sheet that demands a presenting complaint.

"I really don't have any urgent medical needs," I begin, probably with the cockiness of a veteran patient who's been in the trenches too long and thinks he deserves more respect than the new recruits.

Testing the waters further, I continue, as he looks at me quizzically. "I've never been hospitalized with anything AIDS-related, but I don't want to go to my current doctor's hospital. I need to expand my support system."

At this point, it seems timely to offer my neatly typed forms as a kind of peace offering in case he thinks I'm demented, and as evidence of my sincerity.

"Here's all the blood work and a list of the AIDS-related medical problems I've had," I explain, offering the sheets. His eyes sparkle and he says nice things about making his job easier.

Encouraged, I press on. "I need to work with a doctor who will include me in *all* decisions. I need to know *everything*," I emphasize.

After assuring me that I've come to the right place, the gentle assistant excuses himself.

Only then do I test the examination table. After seven years, it seems right to have a few moments alone with it. After all, it was on one of these that I was diagnosed. I touch it, then ease onto the paper-covered vinyl. A knock comes through the door and the doctor enters.

I repeat the little presentation I'd rehearsed on the med tech, adding, "Several of my friends are your patients and the grapevine reviews about you are good."

An electric hum sounds as the chair becomes a table and a hydraulic lift brings it to a convenient height for his probings. By the end of the visit, I discover that he truly does understand my position, my need to be centrally involved with my own case. We've established a dialogue, an understanding.

"Sure, I'll follow you if you like," he says as I pull my pants back on.

Yes, *follow* me is exactly right, I think.

"Thank you." I nod. I mean it.

The elevator shoots me down to the lobby and I strike out into the First Avenue rush hour. Unlike years ago, the colors, noises, and shapes are clearly defined as I sprint down the street.

Excerpts from a Journal

STEPHEN GRECO

26th April 1987

He's gained two pounds—cause for jubilation.

11th May 1987

Ninety, now. He says he can hardly lift an arm without blacking out. I'm scared.

13th May 1987

The white blood cell count now suddenly low.

16th May 1987

His blood pressure sank precipitously this morning, as did his temperature. The nurses found him nearly comatose around dawn, and Rick was with him for three hours before he called

me at noon, to say that if it was another sepsis, as he suspected, then Barry might not be able to last the day. I flew into
the city, wrapped up my baby as only I know how, and flung
myself onto the bed next to him, to keep him warm as I do on
bleak winter nights. Teary, little whispered exchanges, supple-
mented by gentle kisses. And by dinner, the vital signs were
back to normal and Barry was eating. . . .

18th June 1987

Oh, God. Tea with the Ferro-Grumleys, who are just back from
their stay in Rome. After an initial round of cakes and chitchat,
Robert tells me that Michael has just been diagnosed with ARC
and that he, Robert, has KS and has had it for three years. My
dear ones! And the earth changes again. Of course, so much is
clearer now—especially Robert's preoccupation with *Second
Son*, which was bought by Crown just this morning, for a tidy
sum. It will be the first literary book about AIDS and promoted
handsomely as such, Robert says; and the rest of tea was devoted to the problems in making art about AIDS. He stated
plainly the main problem: that writers with AIDS just don't
live long enough to make a book out of their experiences, or
are too exhausted or preoccupied to work efficiently on one. A
damned black hole that swallows our vision. Robert's KS has
been very slow growing and this book—which he says he envisioned, until recently, as his last—has served as an important focus for the past few years of his life. He hasn't told
many people until now, fearing being treated as the "walking
dead," or being interrupted by too much sympathy. But now
that the book will come out, questions of authenticity will
arise—which we debated. I left much later than I'd planned to,
reluctant to leave them but afraid of tiring them further. We sat
in the living room as the afternoon faded, with drops of "Palais
d'Ete" in the air, via a light bulb. Michael, in his robe, man-

aged to be cheery—even to sing a bit of a new song ("Baby Me") from the musical of *Dodsworth* they're perennially working on—despite some pain.

25th June 1987

A small party in the room. Barry's birthday wish: to have a thirty-seventh. At home afterward—having supper alone, watching a bit of *Word Is Out,* which is being broadcast as part of Channel 13's Gay Pride Week Programming—I break down and cry. "God bless us nellie queens. . . ."

30th June 1987

He answered the phone this morning *squealing* in pain. The Hickman catheter had become so infected that his whole side, from the head to the shoulder, was affected. I can handle the bedpans, the injections, and the inevitability of decline, but I found terrifying those pathetic cries. For a moment I froze, then I launched into as soothing a speech as I could manage, trying simultaneously to learn whether Rick had been there yet and whether anyone was doing something. Billy—his roommate—had gone for the nurse, he said; and when I called back later, after leaving a message with Rick, I found that they'd removed the catheter and given Barry a painkiller.

2nd July 1987

A short escape to Sea Girt, thanks to Robert and Michael. Shortly after arriving, I learn (when the first of the afternoon's *two* tea trays is presented) that the boys travel not only with their own sheets—I'd been planning to write about it since they returned from Rome—but their favorite tea cosy as well— the very one in front of me, in fact, which I recognize from their snapshots of the Piazza Monte Vecchio apartment.

3rd July 1987

My tea this morning on the terrace with Robert, who reads parts of *Second Son* to me, including one (about an angry boy dying in the hospitals) that incorporates medical details I rec- ognized from Barry's history.

11th July 1987

He's regressing; there's no other word for it. Though cogent this morning—his message had irony and humor, and was uttered in a strong voice—he was confused when I arrived late in the afternoon, thinking I'd already been there earlier, for lunch. (It was yesterday he was remembering.) He could be home but for this intermittent low-grade fever, which might be the result of some new infection, or of the drug treatment for the last one, or of the underlying HIV infection itself, and which might prevent him from receiving another Hickman catheter.

14th July 1987

The phone rings at eight this morning. It's Barry, in a state, wanting to know why they've just delivered breakfast to his room. He's spent the last hour looking through his menus, trying to come up with a choice for dinner. I am able to reassure him—saying, among other things, that at this time of year, particularly on gray days, the light at seven in the morning looks very much like that at seven at night—but I can't get back to sleep.

4th August 1987

Barry's roommate, Daniel, died early this morning. Ironic, since at last night's care-partner meeting, we discussed Daniel and the effect his increasing needs were having on Barry.

7th August 1987

Barry lost his second roommate last night—this one a boy named Leon, whom we barely got to know, whose mother read to him from the Bible. This morning, the hospital wheeled a VCR into the room for Barry—as sort of a consolation prize, I suppose.

14th August 1987

"I don't like going to these events without you," I told Barry as I was leaving to meet Grahman Lustig at Dance Theater Workshop, for Terry Beck's concert. "I miss hearing what you think about things," I said. Barry smirked, incredulously—probably remembering too many intermission harangues. "Okay," I said, "I miss telling you what you think about things. . . ."

22nd August 1987

Farquhar died last night. I found him curled up under Barry's desk, looking fairly peaceful. Was he lonely, I wonder, with Barry gone and me so preoccupied? Could I have gotten him to the vet weeks ago, despite my mad rushing about among hospital, home, and office? There is no way for me to describe the sadness of that lifeless body, the eeriness of an apartment now free of odors and tracked litter. He was everything to us.

24th August 1987

Barry's home and, with the help of a nurse, doing quite well.

26th August 1987

Still, periods of disorientation. This morning, as Monica, today's nurse, and Joan arrive, he was on to something about closing on an apartment in New Jersey, which I questioned. "I can't sign anything in my pajamas." And in frustration, when my curiosity led me to ask for details: "Oh, Stephen, I'm afraid of winding up someplace that doesn't exist." Last night was calm and I was able to sleep.

1st September 1987

Frequent incontinence.

2nd September 1987

His screams wake me in the middle of the night—he's in pain and scared. His nightmare, of being made some sort of exhibit, supplants mine, about the death of my father.

4th September 1987

It's getting ugly at home. Barry's so confused and contentious that everything becomes an argument. I came back frcm the gym this afternoon to find that he'd barely touched his lunch. We had a long talk, during which I tried everything from sweetness and reason to threats of hospitalization; then I slapped him. It was bitter tears for a while—from both of us— but then the air seemed to clear and I was permitted to make up with him. These scenes take a lot out of me and crop up whether or not a nurse is present; at night they keep me from sleep and during the day they delay my departure for work. This can't go on. . . .

7th September 1987

He's squeezing his cock, kneading it. "Barry, do you want to piss?" I ask. "No," he says. "Barry, are you sure you don't have to piss?" "No, Stephen!" Then I think. "Barry, does anybody have to piss?" And desperately he says, "Yes!" I give him the urinal and out flows a load. We went to twenty-four-hour nursing today and I'm thinking, sadly and with some guilt, about institutional settings. (I find that that word *setting* makes it easier to talk about turning my lover out of the house.) He's become almost unmanageable—refusing food, regularly tearing off his Hickman dressing and disconnecting the Texas catheter, even throwing himself out of bed two or three times a night. (Last night, he did so, I'm told, after ripping off his shirt and waving it like a flag, shouting "I'm at the wrong gate!") And then there's the spinning of endless stories out of threads too mysterious to identify—perhaps overheard conversations, television newscasts, remembered appointments. When you try to understand them, he indefatigably disputes, qualifies, exhorts, grimaces, and involves the other characters—sometimes other Barrys and other Stephens—he seems to have invented to explain or displace his pain. . . .

9th September 1987

The sweet thing about his forgetting exactly who I am, during these awful bouts of dementia, is that he seems to fall in love with me again, fresh, each time I go to comfort him.

16th September 1987

Extremely argumentative today; he wouldn't eat.

20th September 1987

It's over. My dear one died last night at 10:45, with Susan and me at his side. It was peaceful; just what is meant by "a good death," I think—which he specified in his Living Will and asked for again during his final hours, and which we were able to provide for him, *his* gift to us. His pulse and blood pressure had been fading since eight, when the night nurse came on duty; his breathing was labored. I hovered at his left side—half-sitting, half-lying—saying tender words and alternatively wiping his sweaty brow and kissing it; my hand resting protectively over his waist as it did at bedtime during these past fifteen years. Just before the end, he was able to press, weakly but with infinite love that has echoed forth from that moment, his hand over mine. I got up to change the record, but Susan called me back. The rhythm of his breathing was changing, and soon he was gone. We waited until Harriet could arrive before we called Riverside and summoned the police (who were remarkably indelicate). And it was four before the police left, the body was fetched, Harriet and Josh departed, I cleaned up and Susan and I went to bed, numb with exhaustion. Today Jim Saslow stopped by and we planned the memorial service.

21st September 1987

Dressing for the service, I don't find my gold cuff links anywhere and begin to curse one of our nurses. Then the cuff links turn up in the wrong box—where I'd put them, of course—and my paranoia melts into shame. Twenty people had to be turned away from Riverside's door, I was told later. In our innocence, Susan, Harriet, and I had arranged for a room to seat seventy-five—and twice that managed to make it inside. I take the opportunity to see the body for a last time, beforehand.

22nd September 1987

I sit shiva. People visit; I tell and retell the same stories. Vast emptiness, pointlessness. Visiting the hospital every day for eight months was difficult, but it became my joy. Having him home was even harder, but that, too, finally a joy. Now there is nothing, except these inadequate occasions to utter his name.

23rd September 1987

Exhaustion. I nap on the daybed. How much could Barry have seen as he lay dying, I wonder. The basket we brought back from Rangeley two years ago, over which we'd argued bitterly and finally made up—could he see that? At the end, I was whispering that we forgive each other and hoping that the sight of it was a comfort. . . .

25th September 1987

The first time I saw Barry, he was dancing.

1st October 1987

While dressing today, I went to Barry's closet and, with a certain amount of relish, took a tie of his that I helped him buy and have always loved. He sometimes grudgingly let me borrow it. "I'm wearing the Paul Stuart tie! I'm wearing the Paul Stuart tie, and there's nothing you can do about it!" I shouted gleefully, dancing around the apartment, trailing the thing. Then, tying the knot, I knew how handsome he thought me in it—perhaps how handsome I looked to him now, from some cloud—and I wept.

Well, Was It Worth It?

SCOTT TUCKER

Walking through the valley of the shadow of death, many of us are crossing paths with prophets who proclaim either an age-old morality or an up-to-date maturity. We are warned by public figures, both gay and straight, that the sexual revolution is dead, along with so many of the sexual revolutionaries. Some of these prophets are murderously moral, hoping viruses will do the dirty work which bullets, alas, cannot. When Patrick Buchanan, a syndicated columnist and former White House official, discussed the impact of AIDS, he gleefully predicted "the wholesale destruction and scattering of the 'gay communities' of America within several years."

Our own gay prophets are more selective, more benign, but even they are moved by a purging spirit. They preach a gospel of survival through assimilation, which many of us can neither accept nor live by. They would never describe AIDS as the Wrath of God, yet Judeo-Christian moralism is evident in their views of this crisis. AIDS is a flaming sword, and on this Day of Judgment good gays and bad gays will be sorted out, saved or doomed. We must either swim with the moral mainstream or sink beneath it. Good gays can find a place in this society if we play by the rules of marriage and monogamy—and presumably by the rules of adultery and divorce. Bad gays will remain outsiders, identified with promiscuity and plague.

Gay people should be free to choose marriage and monogamy if they wish, but I have no intention of following the most vocal prophets crying out in this wilderness of AIDS. My lover and I have been together over twelve years, and monogamy has not been one of our "marriage bonds." Making a dogma of nonmonogamy is, of course, merely reactive and negative. However, the gay movement is composed of many social and sexual communities, and sexual communalism has been one of many vital bonds between many gay people, both before and after Stonewall. The sexual communalism of gay people deserves a strong defense. Where is such sexual communalism strongest? Among hustlers and porn actors, among drag queens and leatherguys—among all those sexual minorities, in fact, who are stigmatized by the new prophets of old-time religion and of high-tech respectability.

I reached a personal and political milestone during a national lesbian and gay conference in Los Angeles, where debate on topics like pornography and SM had reached a very rowdy pitch. I found myself keeping company with a group of men and women whose political principles and leather finery appealed to me. We formed a "Disgruntled Caucus" and went barhopping one evening, ending up at a packed and steamy bar called The One Way. I'd been to leather bars before, but always like a tourist observing the natives. On that particular night, I saw three knockout bodybuilders enter the bar and perform a ritual that seduced me body and soul. They wore boots, tight jeans, and black leather hoods; their chests were bare and gleaming, lightly oiled and sweaty. Facing each other in a triangle of intimacy and exhibitionism, they drank their beers through their masks and hoods while rubbing and grinding their bodies together. No doubt they lorded their physiques over us mere mortals, but they also graciously accepted the homage we all paid to such brazen beauty. They allowed, even encouraged, the other patrons to take a feel—though I was paralyzed by my own temptation.

Shortly afterward, my lover and I were visiting San Francisco, and a friend zipped me into my new pair of chaps and took me on a tour of the Folsom scene. San Francisco was having one of its rare heat waves, so warm on that night that I was able to wear only a leather harness, while carrying my biker's jacket. In what used to be The Brig, I timidly pressed through the crowd and finally withdrew to a semiquiet corner. In walked a tall, dark, handsome stranger and we made immediate eye contact. He bought me a beer, we talked until I was sure I trusted him, and my initiation into the leather and SM community lasted the rest of that night.

I was entering a sexual community that had been stigmatized long before AIDS; but as that shadow lengthened across the country, and as the death toll grew, leatherfolks were assigned special blame for the spread of the epidemic. Within the gay community, leatherfolk became screens on which danger and temptation were projected, just as gays served the same function for straights at large. It is not surprising that drug abuse, alcoholism, and a degree of irresponsible sexual activity exist in the leather community. But precisely because sexual communalism is a strong element in the leather scene, leatherfolk have also taken great initiative in organizing community events to promote AIDS education and safer sexual practices. In part, this is a natural extension of negotiating sexual roles and limits.

My gravitation toward leatherfolk was certainly sexual, but it was also political and spiritual. As a gay activist, I had grown impatient with conferences and committees, necessary as these often are. Wearing leather is, for me, both a sexual statement and a statement of solidarity with a group which has been shunned and censored even within the gay movement. I also feel that leatherfolk are some of the few people I know who understand the communal and sacramental value of sex. Leatherfolk value privacy, but we insist on our fair share of public space as well. Some of our meetings, whether at campsites or in basements, have a true tribal feeling, and ritual depth. And during a time when so many gay people are in sexual retreat, leatherfolk still glory in the body and varying degrees of sexual drama and exhibitionism.

As the number of the ill and dying increased, I asserted my own body and sexuality more strongly against death. Some would call this narcissism, and so be it. I spent the first months of 1986 working with a construction and renovation crew in Key West, spending my free time at the gym and the beach. I was living a fully physical life for the first time in years, and when I returned home to Philadelphia, I was daring myself to make some changes in my life.

In this risk-taking mood, and feeling tan and fit, I entered a leather contest at a local bar, The Bike Stop. The prize was a trip to Chicago and a chance to compete for the title of International Mr. Leather. I'd seen videos of previous winners—all bulkier and bigger guys than myself—so I was only hoping I'd place among the finalists, and that I'd enjoy the major annual festival of leatherdom. I'm still amused to watch myself win on the video made of the May 1986 contest: I look shell-shocked. But I did collect the bouquet of black leather roses and walk down the ramp into the audience of 1,200 leatherfolk, even managing to pose for photographers while perched on a motorcycle. (A prize I promptly sold, as bicycles have always been more my speed.)

By now, it's a tradition for IML winners to lead a Candlelight March to St. Clement's Church in Chicago for the annual AIDS Memorial Service. I entered the church bedecked in a leather sash big enough for the Jolly Green Giant, on which my new title was emblazoned in studs. Naturally, the leather contingent received a few unfriendly glares, but the ushers thanked us for coming and seated us near the altar.

I lost faith long ago in any omnipotent, benevolent deity; I really find that notion blasphemous, and irreconcilable with a world which is often hellish. Even so, I'm a skeptic with a sense of the sacred, and I was freshly moved when a Mennonite woman whose husband had died of AIDS read from the Book of Job. I'm not sure what the moral of that godawful story may be, but it does resonate in the mind of anyone who tries to make sense of suffering in a time of plague. Later in that service, when a gay choir sang "My Buddy," my quiet tears became open sobs.

People were asked to name aloud anyone close to them who had died of the disease, and then to name those who were living with the disease. I named Sean, a young man living at that time in San Francisco, talented and beautiful, who had been healthy enough to play tennis in the Gay Olympics. One month later, I was riding a float in the San Francisco Gay Pride Parade, dressed in nothing but boots, harness, and a studded leather jock, when we passed a group of hell-fire Fundamentalists carrying a banner reading AIDS IS THE WRATH OF GOD. I bent over and gave them my fullest moon, a moment Sean would have loved—but he was too ill that weekend to attend the festivities. On my last official IML visit to San Francisco, I saw Sean by chance on the sidewalk, and I jumped out of a car to greet him. He was looking as radiant as I'd ever seen him, and that's probably how he most wanted to be remembered. During the last bout of his illness, it seems he only allowed his mother and sister in the hospital room.

Everywhere I went during my travels, a time would always come when someone would draw me aside at some event and say, "I don't know if you heard that Richard died," or "Joe was diagnosed yesterday," or some other piece of news I half-suspected or had long expected. News among leatherfolk can travel from coast to coast faster than small-town gossip over a backyard fence, and we have our share of mean and petty spirits. But our tribalism and nomadism also mean that we often come through with community support when someone is in serious need or in bad health. Many leather and bike club events are fundraisers for AIDS research, for hospices, or even for individuals with special needs.

I don't view AIDS as a blessing in disguise. As William Blake wrote, "Blight never does good to a tree . . . but if it still bear fruit, let none say the fruit was in consequence of the blight." The waves of sentimentalism and moralism are heavy on all sides. In the face of death, some gay people are retreating into the spiritual ether and abandoning the political struggle. Others throw themselves into the struggle, people who could probably use a nice long spell with a guru on a mountaintop. It is natural that AIDS has provoked a crisis in our sexual and spiritual lives; the danger is that gay people will unwittingly accept the moral and political leadership of people who would prefer us back in the closet—or dead.

The walls which we must often break through in order to find other gay people are now being built up again, brick by brick, and not only by people who claim to be our enemies—but also by some folks who claim to be our friends. Gay people are getting some very bad advice from a number of paid professionals who think of themselves as humane but who share a deep-rooted erotophobia. I have in mind a friend who had a tough time coming out as a gay man, despite natural gifts and beauty. Whatever strength he finally gained was undermined by a straight shrink who read him texts on "narcissism" and who advised him to wear clothes which would disguise his fine physique. When my friend was diagnosed with AIDS, the shrink told him that the only safe sex for gay men was no sex. Any alternatives which would allow more pleasure and intimacy—sex toys, fantasy, massage, masturbation, fetishes, rubbers, the proper virus-killing lubricants—went unmentioned. And of course it would never have occurred to this therapist that bondage and SM can be safe sex.

After a full year of travel, of seeing the best and worst of the leatherworld from coast to coast, of riding floats in parades and sitting at bedsides of dying men, I finally passed on the IML title in May 1987, to Thomas Karasch, a sexy and intelligent young West German. On the night following the contest, and following tradition, he led the Candlelight March to St. Clement's. This year, a Tree of Life had been painted on several vertical banners placed in front of the church, and many of us filed forward to inscribe the names of loved ones who had died. I drew a heart around the names of three friends, including Sean, and wrote "At peace" below. I returned to my seat and found myself listening with new ears and new understanding when a woman read Psalm 139. Not the God of synagogues and churches, but the Sacred itself broke like a thunderstorm on my head as this psalm, so familiar from my days at St. Thomas Choir School, worked its magic on me:

> Such knowledge is too wonderful for me; it is so high that I cannot attain to it. Where can I go then from your Spirit? Or where can I flee from your presence? If I climb up to heaven, you art there, if I make the grave my bed, you are there also. . . . If I say, "Surely the darkness will cover me, and the light around me turn to night," Darkness is not dark to you; the night is as bright as the day; darkness and light to you are both alike.

Despite the fact that I remain light-years distanced from organized religion, I do feel that I experienced some powerful visitation of the Holy Spirit, that Spirit which is not only light but also dark, not only heaven but also hell. Much like this world. From this peak, I was dragged down by a reading from Genesis, which was related in no way to the memorial or the real tragedy, and I didn't much care to hear a nice straight Christian passing on God's "Plan for Man," including the advice to be fruitful and multiply. The human race has done so in spades, and any Paradise I care to live in has to make room for queers.

One of the guys who had placed third one year in the IML contest had made a point of calming my case of nerves when the time came for me to compete for my own title. He was a sweet, sexy man with a fine sense of humor, short but well muscled—the type of fellow a friend of mine admiringly calls a "pitzel." His parents are Christians of some crazed, arcane sect, the sort of religionists who flourish like weeds in this dear native soil; and when he revealed to his mother that he'd been diagnosed with AIDS, she gathered up all of heaven's grace and charity into her heart and turned it upon him with this question: "Well, was it worth it?" He's dead now, and the family gave him a proper Christian funeral and burial, to which his deviate and diabolic friends were emphatically not invited.

Well—in the midst of AIDS and looking back on gay life especially since Stonewall—was it worth it? That question looms over many of our personal and political arguments inside and outside the gay movement today. Some folks refer to the sexual revolution as if it had been a misdirected adolescent rebellion from first to last, leaving nothing but disease and death. They even claim a higher morality and a greater maturity.

They did not grow wiser, they just got tired. Certain reactionaries are motivated by envy of the young, and gay people of a younger generation are often too emotionally bruised by the death of friends and lovers to resist such moralism. The sexual revolution will continue despite setbacks, and much of our political work as activists and sexual beings will require patience and persistence. Informing the public about safe sex means challenging censorship—in the schools and in the media. Nor can we negotiate with the government only as gay people acting on our own. On the contrary, AIDS requires us to take a critical look at the entire health-care system, and at the treatment of the poor, racial minorities, prostitutes, prisoners, and drug addicts. Principled coalition politics must be on our agenda.

All such coalitions have this particular danger: In the search for common solutions to common needs, our specific needs and identities are often buried. But if I draw strength from men and women in the leather community—as I do—then I refuse to cut myself off from my own roots and sources. I've mentioned the right-wing prophets who view all lesbian and gay people quite simply as queers, condemned as such. I should state specifically that some of our own gay prophets are drawing their own distinctions between queers and gays, with gays gaining salvation through moral and sexual conformity.

Identity always has a spiritual dimension, and the sexual and social communalism of "queers" will be a genuine force of resistance against reaction. I do not aim to be baptized in the American mainstream, nor to be born again with belief in the higher morality of monogamy. The sex I had years ago in the baths and backrooms remains a source of beauty and power for me, and I bless every man whose body I knew then, and who shared his stories with me. The medical establishment cared little for gay health then, and is showing a belated interest during this deadly epidemic. We are certainly wiser now, but our wisdom owes more to our own struggles than it does to any priest, doctor, or politician.

Mourn the dead, and fight like hell for the living.

Death and the Erotic Imagination

MICHAEL BRONSKI

Sex and death are the two most taboo topics in American culture. Few resources or encouragements exist to deal with either in honest or helpful ways. Yet while both are covered in secrecy or denial, sex and death are relegated to distinctly different social positions. Sex, once unmentionable, is now the basis for endless consumer products and marketing devices. Death, on the other hand, is shunted to the bottom of the agenda, avoided until it can be avoided no more. It is the dirty little secret that calls up euphemisms and embarrassed looks. Death doesn't sell anything, or make us feel better, or even bring up all those "good" guilt feelings that add the zest to sex. Death is always something that happens to other people. We have even invented the categories of "natural" and "unnatural" death, not so much to classify the types of death but to explain it to ourselves; to draw lines as to why it will not happen to us. On some level, everyone knows that death is inevitable, but few people are eager, or equipped, to deal with the fact.

The gay and lesbian liberation movement is very young.

*Many thanks to Cindy Patton and Charley Shively for talking through many of the ideas of this article.

Women and men who were thirty during the Stonewall Riots (and many were much younger) are just now in their late forties. It is no surprise, then, that gay men are having trouble dealing with the huge number of AIDS deaths. The young are never prepared to begin dealing with death—and certainly not the amount of death that has struck the gay male community over the past few years. As of the beginning of 1988, there have been 50,000 cases of AIDS—approximately 37,000 of those have been gay men.

A Death in the Family

Death in this culture has been treated as a personal matter, a family matter. The biological unit pulls closer together, protected by their community, most often centered around a church, and finds way to deal with the loss. Gay men have also done this. Often these gay extended families are stronger, tighter, than nuclear families because they are chosen and built upon mutual support and respect. But these choices and supports do not come easily. In a world that hates homosexuals, these are momentous acts whose strength is seen in their resilience to the myriad pressures against them.

There is very little—and in some case *no*—legal or psychological support from outside the gay community to help deal with those issues. There are no secure legal rights for homosexual lovers, many times no visiting rights for gay friends. By defining "gay" as purely a sexual activity, and a wrong and sinful one at that, the heterosexual world has not allowed itself to see any social, familial, or nurturing aspects of the gay community dealing with death. This should not come as any surprise—nor does it for a gay person—since there is no basic respect for the gay world in which the person with AIDS has lived his life.

It is impossible to be a gay male today and not think of AIDS all the time. Not only are you faced with AIDS every time you read a paper, watch TV, or pick up a magazine—it is there over the morning coffee and just before you go to bed at night—but AIDS is on your mind every time the telephone rings, every time a letter from a slightly distant friend arrives. In Boston, a city not very hard hit by the epidemic, I know of thirty men who have died or been diagnosed. People who live in New York or San Francisco may know as many as forty-five or sixty men who have died or who have AIDS.

THE DISAPPEARED

Because the gay male community is large and loosely knit— made up of groups of friends as well as large socializing networks or bars and baths—a great many people know one another casually or just by sight. It has become commonplace over the last five years to presume that a bar regular may be dying or dead if he is absent for a while. The friendship networks are informal enough that one man might not know whom to ask about a missing man. Often the news of a friend's diagnosis is simply too hard to talk about in the bars or baths the man used to frequent. Sometimes life feels like living under a fascist regime: People just disappear without a word.

Since Stonewall, the gay and lesbian community has established a complex and varied network of newspapers and magazines. But the gay press has not done all that well in helping the community deal with this deluge of death. News coverage of the epidemic has been erratic. While the *New York Native* has been all out in their medical coverage, too often it is presented in an alarmist, noninformative manner, not very useful for readers who are dealing with their own personal hysterias. *Gay Community News*, on the other hand, has had a tacit policy of not covering medical news, and while they have done some good work about public-policy issues, they have not even printed safe-sex guidelines in the past three years. On the more personal level, both papers will print obits of somewhat prominent people—those who may have been known by some segments of the gay community. While this personalizes the effect of AIDS in a tangible manner, it also isolates and diminishes the number of cases. This practice also implies, however unintentionally, that these cases are sadder because the men were well known, or because they made some contribution to the gay community while they were alive. This is a comfort to many readers who feel that these few isolated cases—not even the tip of the iceberg—portend no warning to their own lives. The most extreme case is, of course, Rock Hudson, who while he never came out, even on his deathbed, still garnered publicity and sympathy simply for being famous.

READING THE OBITS

Other papers, like *The Bay Area Reporter* in San Francisco, run anywhere from ten to twenty obituaries every week of regular, everyday gay men who have died of AIDS. This is a chilling sight, a regular memento mori, especially since many people first see the paper in bars and other gay establishments where it is given away. Reading *BAR* is like walking through a graveyard, or viewing the Vietnam Veterans' Memorial Wall—the only difference is that you knew these people and may have seen them only a week ago. The ultimate effect is to bring the war home; there is no way for a gay man to look at those pages of postage-sized, black-framed portraits and not have some presentiment that this could have been him. And might be in several months' time.

Of course, the straight press is still worse. *The New York Times* will infrequently acknowledge an AIDS-related death as such, usually dependent upon the family, or friends, of the deceased not trying to suppress the fact. Or, in a homophobic reversal of this, the media uses AIDS as one more attack upon the dead person, as the *Times* did in the obit of Roy Cohn. But even when AIDS isn't mentioned, figuring out who is gay and who died of the syndrome is easy: He was thirty-six, a church organist, and died after a short illness, leaving parents and a brother in Connecticut; he was forty-two, a respected clothing designer, died after a long illness, leaving a mother and two sisters in Ohio. But these are just the more prominent, the semifamous by *The New York Times* standards. There is no mention of the thirty-seven-year-old underwriter for an insurance company who died after being hospitalized for eight months, leaving no family because they have not spoken to him since he moved from upstate New York eighteen years ago after telling them he was gay. Nor was AIDS cited in the extensive obituaries of a Boston Latino community leader who died of respiratory complications at the age of thirty-five last spring. Every time one of these obituaries appears, not only AIDS is rendered invisible but also the existence of all gay people.

A startling sense of déjà vu occurs for gay men and lesbians when they read each of these obituaries. It is not unlike twenty years ago when you read gossip columns and newspaper items to see who was married and who was not in order to discover who might be gay and who might (with good reason) be hiding their sexuality. You read these things in an attempt to get a sense of community, to find others who were like you, to feel not so invisible and alone. The social embarrassment and denial of gay sexuality in the 1950s and 1960s is being reenacted now in both the gay and straight worlds by the embarrassment and denial of death and AIDS.

DEATH AND THE TERRITORY—MOVEMENTS AND MARTYRS

The gay community's dealing with death did not begin with AIDS. Before the advent of AIDS, the deaths of young gay men I knew were from queer-bashing. Gay men and lesbians knew that the risks of transgressing heterosexual limits could be dangerous. In both rural and urban areas, in even the most sophisticated, open cities, a gay man or lesbian can be spotted as a homosexual and queer-bashed—and not just beaten but murdered. In the summer of 1986, there were six known gay murders and countless queer-bashings in Boston alone. (And remember, not even the most flagrant heterosexuals are beaten just because they are heterosexuals.) For many, the connections between death and being gay are very clear. If you were "obvious," if you were "known," if you were seen leaving a gay bar, you could be beaten and killed. Death, as it were, came with the territory.

But in some way, this ever-present death was, while hard to deal with, clear in its origins. Death was one more form of oppression that occurred because of homophobia—or in less euphemistic terms—because people hated queers. These deaths were part of the social reality that spawned the gay and lesbian liberation movement. Lesbians and gay men learned to deal with these deaths by taking their cues from other, more established social-activist movements. On the one hand, the dead were seen as martyrs to the "cause." This is clear in the case of Charlie Howard—an effeminate gay man who was murdered by street thugs in Bangor, Maine: There are yearly memorials to him and both legal reform and educational organizing are done in his name. This is not all that different from leftists and labor organizers using the names of images of Joe Hill, Frank Little, and Wesley Everest, as well as the victims of the Triangle Shirtwaist Factory fire and those killed in the Ludlow massacre and the Haymarket riot hangings. The two most famous quotes in activist folklore are Joe Hill's "Don't mourn, organize" and Mother Jones's "Pray for the dead, but fight like hell for the living." Although the latter makes a nod at acknowledging the dead, both place the emphasis on more immediate political action. These were clearly a response to a cultural inclination to sentimentality (based, in part, on a strain of Christianity), which attempted to secure the status quo by keeping people's minds off the present, by keeping them on the past. In the real world, the material world, tending to the aftereffects, the psychological aftershock of death came second to organizing and preparing for the future. The Left has not been able to deal with AIDS in part due to its homophobia, but also because they have always made death a class issue: who was drafted to fight in Vietnam, who is denied health care and proper social services, who is at risk in the workplace. But AIDS cuts across class lines, as well as political lines (it is hard to come up with any sympathy for Roy Cohn, yet he is as much a victim of AIDS as anyone else).

POLITICIZING DEATH

Since AIDS has become recognized as a problem affecting gay men, the community has done an amazing job of mobilization. There are health crises centers, AIDS Action Committees, support systems, and direct service groups, all made up almost entirely by gay men, and to a lesser degree by lesbians, with very little help—until recently—from the heterosexual world. To see what gay men have done in such a short period of time is staggering. But what has been done is in the tradition of most of the work in the gay movement—a direct response to an oppressive situation. Gay men were literally dying in the streets and they were taken in. Gay men were being evicted from their homes, fired from their jobs, denied basic health rights: All of these problems were faced head-on.

But the gay movement has only begun to deal with the psychological response to AIDS and to death. We have not been faced with this much death—this close to home—ever before. The gay community, both men and women, is beginning to realize that there is no more business as usual. The more profound, lasting, and deep repercussions of AIDS are just beginning to be felt. They will not become really evident for another few years and will last for years and years after that. Every day that we do not deal with our feelings and reality, we will have to do so threefold in the future. In many ways, the gay community has followed two of the most traditional responses to death: terror and pity. You can see these enacted in gay men's lives and in any number of popular books or magazines.

The first is the phobic response. A reaction to fear and terror. Some gay men have avoided sex, avoided bars, avoided dealing with their basic sexual identity. Equating gay life with AIDS, and hence with death, they have turned their backs on it. They are filled with fear and loathing for their past lives and their current sexual desires—not a surprising reaction, since this is the lesson that every homosexual has been taught since birth. Sometimes it takes very extreme forms, such as deciding to be heterosexual and to marry, removing one's self from the gay world completely. Other times, a more moderate form of denial occurs, such as joining Sex Addicts Anonymous in an attempt to get one's "dangerous behavior" under control. But what is even more common is a self-conscious self-removal from the active gay world: stop going out to bars, cut down on the amount of energy one might have put into socializing, sometimes even avoiding the gay press because it is "too depressing." All of these reactions are understandable. AIDS *is* too difficult to think about. But each of these responses is not only an avoidance of AIDS—it is also a denial and a whittling away at the gay community; a slow process that—unless we can find a way to combat it—may have a lasting, disastrous effect on the community itself.

The second traditional response—pity—is seen as sentimentality. You see this attitude in all those articles in major magazines about people with AIDS: It is such a shame they are dying because they had such great careers, such wonderful lives, such beautiful apartments, such well-developed bodies. There is nothing facetious here. Almost every piece that appeared in pre-1987 *Life, Time, Look,* and *Newsweek* was certain to mention the tasteful, well-decorated apartments. Compare these articles to the news and features on people of color and AIDS and how their tenement, slum surroundings are the perfect accompaniment—not ironic juxtaposition—to their disease.

Many gay men had a positive response to these pieces, and looking for the sympathy vote is an easy trap for gay men to fall into, because it seems to address oppression: "You may have hated us, but now since we are dying, you have to like us." Such thinking, of course, is false consciousness, because people who hate queers are probably *glad* we are dying—and will take the opportunity to blame us for "spreading" it to the straights. Such thinking adds to the notion that AIDS is a gay disease and reinforces the idea that it is a metaphor for gay life itself.

This whole tradition fits neatly into an old, ingrained, Western cultural tradition, the Camille syndrome: the romance of the outlaw, the misunderstood one who may die, but who dies beautifully and with a great deal of pathos and sentiment. Here is the ultimate incurable romantic.

Anyone who has seen a person die of AIDS knows that this disease is not romantic. There are tubes and respirators, open sores and lesions, inflated and cooled mattresses to keep the fevers down to a manageable 103 degrees, balding due to chemotherapy, infections that coat the mouth and make it impossible to eat. Men who were once 200 pounds lie in bed reduced to 110-pound skeletons. Faces once brimming with life and lust are reduced to courageous death masks animated only with the desire to live.

Because of AIDS, the gay community is now going to have to begin dealing with death in a manner that speaks to both the mind and the spirit: to social actions and emotions. The effects of AIDS are going to be measured not only in the number of deaths but also in the psychological and emotional ravages on the community, in the feelings of rage, impotence, unresolved emotions, and outright terror visited on gay men. The questions raised by this reality range from the obvious "How do you deal with this amount of personal, communal, and political loss?" to the more pressing, and for many more paramount, "How do you have sex when everyone around you is dying?"

The first step in this is to bring death out into the open. Not to avoid talking about it and hiding it as though death was a dirty little secret. There is nothing romantic, nothing sentimental—not even anything *more* frightening—about dying of AIDS. It is not, as Susan Sontag might point out, a metaphor for anything. It is like all death: a painful hard end to the painful and sometimes hard act of living.

RADICALIZING SEX
SEX AS METAPHOR
DEATH AND THE EROTIC IMAGINATION

Between sex and death, gay people have dealt very well with sexual pleasure. We have liberated sex from the confines of the state and religion, from the proscriptions of gender, and have legitimized unadulterated sexual pleasure—purely creative, not procreative—as an end unto itself. It is a message that has been heeded by the rest of the world as well. As gay people, we have to learn to deal with death in the way that we have learned to deal with sex. To see it for what it is and to view it realistically. And along with this, we have to try to understand its effect on us, and to acknowledge the place of grief and mourning in our lives.

Up until now, the gay movement has learned—partly from the Left and partly from our own organizing—to radicalize death: to use death as an impetus for social change. The deaths of Joe Hill, Charlie Howard, and all of the men with AIDS have been an incentive to move forward and to change society. What we are faced with doing now—in the wake of so much death, so much inconsolation—is to politicize death, to bring it into our whole lives and to understand all of its implications for us, both social and personal, to make death part of a seamless web of existence neither avoided nor sentimentalized.

Conversely, we have learned to politicize sex, to bring sexual desire into our full lives and to meld the personal and the political together. From the second wave of feminism (as well as from gay male writers from Oscar Wilde to Tennessee Williams), we have learned to see the connections between sex and politics. There is a strong link—a physical one if you believe in the usually acknowledged routes of HIV transmission—between sex and death. We have to face that connection. If we are to face it without fear, we must radicalize sex as we did death. Sift through the cultural mythologies and trappings we attach to sexuality, and try to reimagine it. Education around AIDS will help create this vision, but we also have to look in ourselves and understand what sex means to us—and what we have allowed it to mean in this homophobic culture.

One of the main differences between AIDS organizing and other political organizing is that many of the people who are doing the groundwork are at high risk—some at very high risk—for the disease. There is no need—as they used to say—to bring the war home: It is here already. It is here in the number of AIDS deaths, in the untold (and continually uncounted) numbers of suicides, and in the emotional deaths many gay men are suffering.

The gay movement can learn to deal with death in the same way it has learned to deal with sex: not as a means to an end, as a metaphor, but as a physical experience, a material, not a moral, reality. There is no inherent mystery surrounding sex and death—those myths are purely social inventions to control behavior and make us conform to certain mores and standards. Sex and death are part of life, and the metaphors, the allegories, the fears, and the fallacies that have been built up around them were invented to keep us from enjoying life and facing death without fear.

The Bible tells us that the wages of sin are death. But the

reality is that everyone dies, regardless of sin. Our traditions tell us that death is payment for transgressions. As long as we believe somewhere that sex leads to death, it will be impossible to view AIDS without moralizing and mystifying it.

In the past year, there have been some moves to deal with the grief, the loss, the incalculable hurt that AIDS has caused the gay community. The NAMES Project Quilt—which is now traveling around the country—seems to be not only a concrete memorial but a way for all of us to acknowledge and deal with our own pain, as well as a call to action.

No one, except, perhaps, those who choose suicide, wants to die and certainly no one wants to die of AIDS. We as gay people must learn to face the reality of death with the same energy and imagination we have put into claiming and enjoying our sexual desires and experiences. When we do not deal with death, it will continue to cause us more stress, more hurt, and more self-doubt. It will be used as another weapon against us—used to deny us ourselves. When death—like sex—remains taboo, clouded behind moralism, abstractions, sentimentality, fear, and inadequate notions of politics, we will not be able to claim it as another aspect of our openly gay lives.

Esthetics and Loss

EDMUND WHITE

I had a friend, a painter named Kris Johnson, who died two years ago of AIDS. He was in his early thirties. He'd shown here and there, in bookstores, arty coffee shops, that kind of thing, first in Minnesota, then in Los Angeles. He painted over color photos he'd color-Xeroxed—images of shopping carts in parking lots, of giant palms, their small heads black as warts against the smoggy sun: California images.

He read *Artform* religiously; he would have been happy to see his name in its pages. The magazine represented for him a lien on his future, a promise of the serious work he was about to embrace as soon as he could get out of the fast lane. Like many people who are both beautiful and gifted, he had to explore his beauty before his gift. It dictated his way of living until two years ago, before his death. His health had already begun to deteriorate and he'd moved to Santa Fe, where he painted seriously his last few months.

By now there have been many articles about how the AIDS virus is contracted and how it manifests itself. The purely medical horrors of the disease have received the attention of the world press. What interests me here is how artists of all sorts—writers, painters, sculptors, people in video and performance art, actors, models—are responding to AIDS in their work and their lives. If I narrow the focus, I do so because of the impact the epidemic has had on esthetics and on the life of the art community, an impact that has not been studied.

The most visible artistic expressions of AIDS have been movies, television dramas, and melodramas on the stage, almost all of which have emphasized that AIDS is a terribly moving human experience (for the lover, the nurse, the family, the patient), which may precipitate the coming out of the doctor (the play *Anti Body*, 1983, by Louise Parker Kelley) or overcome the homophobia of the straight male nurse (*Compromised Immunity*, 1986, by Andy Kirby and the Gay Sweatshop Theatre Company, from England) or resolve long-standing tensions between lovers (William M. Hoffman's play *As Is*, 1985, and Bill Sherwood's beautifully rendered movie *Parting Glances*, 1985). Although Larry Kramer's play *The Normal Heart*, 1985, is almost alone in taking up the political aspects of the disease, it still ends in true melodramatic fashion with a deathbed wedding scene. John Erman's *An Early Frost*, 1985, a made-for-television movie on NBC, is the *Love Story* of the eighties; the best documentary is perhaps *Coming of Age*, 1986, by Marc Huestis, who filmed scenes from the life of a friend of his diagnosed with the virus.

But even on artists working away from the limelight, AIDS has had an effect. Naturally the prospect of ill health and death or its actuality inspires a sense of urgency. What was it I wanted to do in my work after all? Should I make my work simpler, clearer, more accessible? Should I record my fears obliquely or directly, or should I defy them? Is it more heroic to drop whatever I was doing and look disease in the eye or should I continue going in the same direction as before, though with a new consecration? Is it a hateful concession to the disease even to acknowledge its existence? Should I pretend Olympian indifference to it? Or should I admit to myself, "Look, kid, you're scared shitless and that's your material"? If sex and death are the only two topics worthy of adult consideration, then AIDS wins hands down as subject matter.

It seems to me that AIDS is tilting energies away from the popular arts (including disco dancing, the sculpturing of the living body through working out, the design of pleasure machines—bars, clubs, baths, resort houses) and redirecting them toward the solitary "high" arts. Of course I may simply be confusing the effects of aging with the effects of the disease; after all, the Stonewall generation is now middle-aged, and older people naturally seek out different pursuits. But we know how frightened everyone is becoming, even well beyond the "high risk" group that is my paradigm and my subject here.

What seems unquestionable is that ten years ago sex was a main reason for being for many gay men. Not simple, humdrum coupling, but a new principle of adhesiveness. Sex provided a daily brush with the ecstatic, a rehearsal of forgotten pain under the sign of the miraculous—sex was a force binding familiar atoms into new polymers of affinity.

To be sure, as some wit once remarked, life would be supportable without its pleasures, and certainly a sensual career had its melancholy side. Even so, sex was if not fulfilling then at least engrossing—enough at times to make the pursuit of the toughest artistic goals seem too hard, too much work given the mild returns. "Beauty is difficult," as Pound liked to remind us, and the difficulties held little allure for people who could take satisfaction in an everyday life that had, literally, become . . . sensational. Popular expressions of the art of life, or rather those pleasures that intensified the already heady exchange within a newly liberated culture, thrived: the fortune that was lavished on flowers, drugs, sound systems, food, clothes, hair. People who were oppressed by the brutality of the big city or by their own poverty or a humiliating job could create for at least a night, or a weekend, a magical dreamlike environment.

Now all that has changed. I, for one, at least feel repatriated to my lonely adolescence, the time when I was alone with my writing and I felt weird about being a queer. Art was a consolation then—a consolation for a life not much worth living, a site for the staging of fantasies reality couldn't fulfill, a peopling of solitude—and art has become a consolation again. People aren't on the prowl anymore, and a seductive environment is read not as an enticement but as a death trap. Fat is in; it means you're not dying, at least not yet.

And of course we do feel weird again, despised, alien. There's talk of tattooing us or quarantining us. Both the medical and the moralistic models for homosexuality have been dusted off only fifteen years after they were shelved; the smell of the madhouse and the punitive vision of the Rake Chastised have been trotted out once more. In such a social climate, the popular arts, the public arts, are standing still, frozen in time. There's no market, no confidence, no money. The brassy hedonism of a few years back has given way to a protective gray invisibility, which struck me forcibly when I returned to New York recently after being away for several months. As Joe Orton in his diary quotes a friend remarking, all we see are all those dull norms, all norming about.

But if the conditions for a popular culture are deteriorating, those promoting a renewed high culture have returned. Certainly the disease is encouraging homosexuals to question whether they want to go on defining themselves at all by their sexuality. Maybe the French philosopher Michel Foucault was right in saying there are homosexual acts but not homosexual people. More concretely, when a society based on sex and expression is deeroticized, its very reason for being can vanish.

Yet the disease is a stigma; even the horde of asymptomatic carriers of the antibody is stigmatized. Whether imposed or chosen, gay identity is still very much with us. How does it express itself these days?

The main feeling is one of evanescence. It's just like the Middle Ages; every time you say goodbye to a friend, you fear it may be for the last time. You search your own body for signs of the malady. Every time someone begins a sentence with

"Do you remember Bob . . ." you seize up in anticipation of the sequel. A writer or visual artist responds to this fragility as both a theme and as a practical limitation—no more projects that require five years to finish.

The body becomes central, the body that until recently was at once so natural (athletic, young, casually dressed) and so artificial (pumped up, pierced, ornamented). Now it is feeble, yellowing, infected—or boisterously healthy as a denial of precisely this possibility. When I saw a famous gay filmmaker recently, he was radiant, with a hired tan; "I have to look healthy or no one will bankroll me." Most of all the body is unloved. Onanism—singular or in groups—has replaced intercourse. This solitude is precisely a recollection of adolescence. Unloved, the body releases its old sad song, but it also builds fantasies, rerunning idealized movies of past realities, fashioning new images out of thin air.

People think about the machinery of the body—the wheezing bellows of the lungs, the mulcher of the gut—and of the enemy it may be harboring. "In the midst of life we are in death," in the words of the Book of Common Prayer. Death—in its submicroscopic, viral, paranoid aspect, the side worthy of William Burroughs—shadows every pleasure.

The New York painter Frank Moore told me last fall that in developing possible sets and costumes for a new Lar Lubovitch ballet, he worked out an imagery of blood cells and invading organisms, of cells consuming themselves—a vision of cellular holocaust. In his view, the fact of death and the ever-present threat of mortality have added a bite to the sometimes empty rhetoric of East Village expressionism. "Until now anger has been a look, a pose," he told me. Now it has teeth.

The list of people in the art world who have died of AIDS is long and growing longer. I won't mention names for fear of omitting one—or including one that discretion should conceal (it's not always possible to verify how much a patient told his family).

Maybe it's tactless or irrelevant to critical evaluation to consider an artist, writer, dealer, or curator in the light of his death.

Yet the urge to memorialize the dead, to honor their lives, is a pressing instinct. Ross Bleckner's paintings with titles such as *Hospital Room, Memoriam,* and *8,122 + As of January, 1986* commemorate those who had died of AIDS, and incorporate trophies, banners, flowers, and gates—public images.

There is an equally strong urge to record one's own past—one's own life—before it vanishes. I suppose everyone both believes and chooses to ignore that each detail of our behavior is inscribed in the arbitrariness of history. Which culture, which moment we live in determines how we have sex, go mad, marry, die, and worship, even how we say Ai! instead of Ouch! when we're pinched. Not even the soul that we reform or express is God-given or eternal; as Foucault writes in *Discipline and Punish* (1978), "The soul is the effect and instrument of a political anatomy; the soul is the prison of the body." For gay men this force of history has been made to come clean; it's been stripped of its natural look. The very rapidity of change has laid bare the clanking machinery of history. To have been oppressed in the fifties, freed in the sixties, exalted in the seventies, and wiped out in the eighties is a quick itinerary for a whole culture to follow. For we are witnessing not just the death of individuals but a menace to an entire culture. All the more reason to bear witness to the cultural moment.

Art must compete with (rectify, purge) the media, which has thoroughly politicized AIDS in a process that is the subject of a book to be published shortly in England. It is *Policing Desire: Pornography, AIDS and the Media* by Simon Watney. (Watney, Jeffrey Weeks, Richard Goldstein, and Dennis Altman rank as the leading English-language intellectuals to think about AIDS and homosexuality.)

This winter William Olander at the New Museum in New York has organized "Homo Video—Where We Are Now," an international gay and lesbian program that focuses in part on AIDS and the media. For instance, Gregg Bordowitz's *". . . some aspect of a shared lifestyle,"* deals with the contrast between the actual diseases and the "gay plague" image promoted by the media. John Greyson's, *Moscow Does Not Believe in Queers*, 1986, inserts lurid Rock Hudson headlines into a taped diary of ten days at a 1985 Moscow youth festival where Greyson functioned as an "out" homosexual in a country that does not acknowledge the rights—or even the legitimate existence—of homosexuals. And Stuart Marshall's *Bright Eyes*, 1986, tracks, among other things, the presentation of AIDS in the English media.

If art is to confront AIDS more honestly than the media has done, it must begin in tact, avoid humor, and end in anger.

Begin in tact, I say, because we must not reduce individuals to their deaths; we must not fall into the trap of replacing the afterlife with the moment of dying. How someone dies says nothing about how he lived. And tact because we must not let the disease stand for other things. AIDS generates complex and harrowing reflections, but it is not caused by moral or intellectual choices. We are witnessing at long last the end of illness as metaphor and metonym.

Avoid humor, because humor seems grotesquely inappropriate to the occasion. Humor puts the public (indifferent when not uneasy) on cosy terms with what is an unspeakable scandal: death. Humor domesticates terror, lays to rest misgivings that should be intensified. Humor suggests that AIDS is just another calamity to befall Mother Camp, whereas in truth AIDS is not one more item in a sequence, but a rupture in meaning itself. Humor, like melodrama, is an assertion of bourgeois values; it falsely suggests that AIDS is all in the family. Baudelaire reminded us that the wise man laughs only with fear and trembling.

End in anger, I say, because it is only sane to rage against the dying of the light, because strategically anger is a political response, because psychologically anger replaces despondency, and because existentially anger lightens the solitude of frightened individuals.

I feel very alone with the disease. My friends are dying. One of them asked me to say a prayer for us all in Venice "in that church they built when the city was spared from the ravages of the plague." Atheist that I am, I murmured my invocation to Longhena's Baroque octagon if not to any spirit dwelling in Santa Maria della Salute. The other day I saw stenciled on a Paris wall an erect penis, its dimensions included in centimeters, and the words *Faut Pas Rever* (You mustn't dream). When people's dreams are withdrawn, they get real angry, real fast.

The NAMES Project

ROBERT DAWIDOFF

1. Remembrance. History and art and the stories the old tell the young and the young think are important enough to remember to tell when they grow old. It's just the things that matter enough in life to repeat and pass on. This is as old as human civilization. It is what we do. We tell others for whom we care what we have learned about life. That's what The NAMES Project is. It is a collection of some very important things its creators have learned about life. Some things worth remembering, some things important to pass along.

2. Names. If you look at the stories of any civilization you will find lots of names. The names of people we never knew crowd our memories and say something to us. Think of the names we all know, Solomon and Hamlet and Mary and Ulysses and Cleopatra and Babe Ruth and Marie Antoinette. Each name brings something to mind, a quality; Solomon's wisdom, a dilemma; Hamlet's indecisiveness; a spiritual state, Mary's blessed motherhood; an adventure, Ulysses's journey home; the fatal charms of Cleopatra; the slugging of the Babe; the indifference of Marie Antoinette to the world around her. The names remind us of what life is all about. That is why we remember them too, because generations of human beings have

recognized that there was something special about those
names because of what their lives remind us to think about.

3. Of course, the names we know best are the names of our
friends and family, the people who keep us company in life
and who make it bearable and worth living, the names of the
people we have loved, and the names we remember because
we miss them when they die, as they would miss us. After
shock and grief and even anger, when we lose someone we
love, we can remember them by naming them and conjuring
them up inside us. We keep mementos of them, things our
parents gave us, dried up flowers and old photographs and
some ribbons or a party favor, stories of our lives with family
and friends, memories of the good times and bad. Our memories can be triggered and our feelings rekindled by the least
memento, something dear to that person, and most of all by
the name. We seldom stop to think of all that *is* in a name. Say
the name of someone you love and whom you miss, and what
you loved and what you miss comes flooding back into your
heart.

4. Where the names belong. Sometimes we carve the names on
a stone, sometimes we paint pictures of them, sometimes we
write them down. Sometimes we try to forget them. Sometimes we erect statues to make sure people remember the
names, sometimes we make prayers of the names of the dead.
The NAMES Project tries to do all these things for those who
have died of AIDS. The large Quilt gives vibrant testimony to
the lives of the people who have died of AIDS by tapping the
memories of those who miss them.

5. The originators of The NAMES Project did something as old
as time and American as apple pie. Human beings have always

taken to the loom and the stitch when they wanted to honor life. Americans have quilted from the start. The idea was to pass along to the generations something useful and beautiful, something to warm the outer and the inner being. From the start, the Quilt had patterns that symbolized the meaning of life, the joys and sorrows and the special memories of the family, cherished names and pictures and pieces of life.

6. The NAMES Project is made up of thousands of panels in which the lives of people who have died of AIDS are remembered and illuminated in the colors and fabrics and shapes and objects and words, the pictures and textures and qualities, that made them special. Like people from the beginning of time, the contributors to The NAMES Project have used art and love to keep the spirit of their loved ones alive. Like a memorial, therefore, the Quilt is a powerful experience of human life and feeling.

Graveyards are gloomy but memorials are not. Most of art is remembrance. And The NAMES Project is not a traveling cemetery or even a war memorial. The Quilt thrills with the lives of human beings it memorializes. Each single panel is made up of grief and memory and love and anger and hope. Each panel gives us the life of a person rendered in art from the stuff of lives and the fabrics of feelings. It is about the life the person lived and the impact that life had on others.

7. The experience of the Quilt is overwhelming. It is not like visiting a place or viewing something, it is being in the Quilt, as if enfolded by it. You go to look and suddenly the Quilt makes you present in your own life because of the surrounding atmosphere of lives, lives, lives. . . . You experience it by walking up and down and around the aisles from which the thousands of panels are all accessible to view. At first, you are stunned by the number of the panels, almost overwhelmed at

first by the fact of the human cost of this frightful disease. You stand back for a moment, with the toll in human lives AIDS has taken suddenly right there, before you. Anything particular dims in this grim reality. It is powerful and scary and shocking.

Then from your own horror of death, the panels draw you back into life. They give individuality and color and reality back to the ungraspable mystery. As you wander through the aisles, your eye is caught by this or that panel, the way in life our eyes and hearts are caught by this or that person. For the time you spend in the country of the Quilt, you experience what it is like to live with all these persons, the emotions that their lives bring out in you are elicited by the extraordinary variety and interest of the panels. The Quilt provides a participatory experience of human creativity.

8. Like something out of Walt Whitman, The NAMES Project gives us the multitude of individuals in a collective democracy; their individual lives glow with color against the democracy of death. What is so arresting about this memorial is that most of the toll of AIDS is on the young and the Quilt reminds us of the heroic beauty and the desperate pathos and the renewed sense of the meaning of life bequeathed to their survivors by those who die too young. The terrifying thing about AIDS is that it brings into almost every American life the experience of that loss, a generation of talented creative people, sons, daughters, sisters, brothers, parents, children, uncles, aunts, cousins, friends, citizens, a collection of startling individual human lives caught in midflight and preserved for all time by this Quilt. The Quilt does not suggest a single meaning to death except perhaps that in the way the remembered lived we can find out about what makes life worth living and worth fighting for and worth honoring when it is left too soon and needlessly.

*   *   *

9. The NAMES Project is so various and works such a human magic on our feelings as we participate in it that it melts the iceberg of feeling that has encased America's reaction to AIDS and sets the waters of human feeling free to flow again. It breaks the silence once and for all and 'changes fear into feeling. The experience of the Quilt is one of exquisite cathartic relief, enabling relief, comfort and community and emotion. The silence is broken when we hear our hearts speaking to us as we bear witness to the lives lost to AIDS. The NAMES Project gives us hope because you can't know what to do until you know how you feel. And The NAMES Project is reminding Americans in the most human, expressive way of how we really feel about one another and therefore what we must do about it.

10. Of course, AIDS has taken every kind of life, male, female, young, old, child, adult; every kind of person has died of AIDS. The NAMES Project reminds us of that. A child's bed strewn with her stuffed animals remembers a little girl. But, as everyone knows, gay men have been especially hard hit by AIDS. The NAMES Project is, among other things, a remarkable, living record of the recent history of gay Americans. The panels unfold a story of love, friendship, creativity, and human worth that chokes the viewer with pride and sadness. In the midst of this catastrophe, The NAMES Project stands up for the lives gay men enjoyed and defends the dead from slurs and dishonor. It is impossible to see the panels without feeling a new respect and kinship and connection with these men. And the community of concern and love that extends from each panel outward to friends and family makes a powerful political point that death is not what gay life or love is about and that the accomplishments of the gay movement must not

be sacrificed along with so many lives to this disease and that the dreams these panels remind us of, the human dreams of so many gay men, are now ours to dream for them, as well as for ourselves.

The NAMES Project is like a history lesson. Some names still, anonymous, closeted the way so many of us have had to live, some elaborate in their public gayness. AIDS is not a gay disease. But AIDS is a terrible fact of gay history. The NAMES Project records that history and in itself is a testimony to the brave, stubborn, funny, beautiful, human, loving community of gay men and their lesbian sisters and their friends and loved ones. AIDS is not only happening to gays, let alone to gay men, but it is happening to them and The NAMES Project is an extraordinary tribute to and by and for a community under desperate, unlooked for, unmerited siege. The NAMES Project holds up a mirror to gay life and the full beautiful constructive humanity of our community shines back at us. The NAMES Project holds up a mirror to every human being who cares to look. It reflects the best, the noblest human qualities that come out in the harshest human conditions.

11. Some panels. Chaz's silver white dress, a weeping golden sun shining on "unknown," a rainbow of colors for Provincetown anonymous, George Kit Zoll "the resting rainbow," "sweet dreams," butterflies for Ahmed Hernandez. John Conley of San Francisco made a panel of an airmail letter with a teddy bear stamp addressed to "Mark Richer, A Better Place." A black and white panel memorializing several "black and white men together," pink and green linked flowers of the linked lives and deaths of two lovers, Charles Ludlam memorialized in a wonderful portrait as Camille, symbols of peace and love and rainbows and portraits of the dead, and then in the midst of all this loving remembrance "Roy Cohn: Bully, Coward, Victim." Tom B. with beadspreads, little hearts, and a

funny nose, Richard Sand with little Pooh bears embroidered and the legend "hug me," Charlie's name in red across a bull, memorialized by his friends, the philosopher Michel Foucault with one of his statements. Below Foucault's panel, signatures on pink satin of the friends of a mourned friend. They go on; a child's bed, an artist's work, Rock Hudson, a friend's favorite things. . . .

12. The other thing in The NAMES Project is the other people there seeing it with you. Being with lots of people is not always the key to thinking well of one's fellow human creatures. Being with the other people at the Quilt is part of its blessing. In the collection of the panels and all the responses we share to it is the community of hope that folk art makes from grief so that people can go on . . . together.

More than anything else, the experience of the Quilt is one of community with other people, the other ones right there with you, right then. You can't help recognizing the emotions they are having, the same ones, the different ones, and your being human with the capacity to feel and express is something the naming of the names of the dead reminds us of.

You leave The NAMES Project with a deeper sense of yourself and a deeper sense of your kind, the human community of life and death, of shared joy and suffering. The NAMES Project is more than a memorial, more than folk art, more than fundraising, more even than the all-encompassing fight against AIDS. It is a rare and intense experience in what it means to be human. The community that has had to cope with AIDS, the PWAs, the lovers and families and friends and health workers and volunteers and scientists, everyone who has been busy with this disease, have made in this Quilt a generous gift to all of us.

The Quilt gives us our most direct feelings back, our feelings of belonging, our sense of the precariousness of life and why it is worth clinging to, how it can be lived and how tragically it can be lost and how beautifully, after all, it can be relinquished and how vibrantly it can be remembered. In the moment of self-recognition—*I am a human being, frail and strong, lucky and unlucky*—the visitor to The NAMES Project makes the connection between self and others that is where the fight against AIDS must be constantly refreshed.

You will feel the grief and the anger, the loss and admiration, the determination to end this disease because The NAMES Project makes it real, a part of your life, not just someone else's death.

AIDS, Art and Obits

MICHAEL BRONSKI

Peter Hujar	1934–1987
Choo San Goh	1948–1987
Gerald Chapman	1950–1987
Barry Laine	1951–1987
Jerry Carlson	1956–1987

I was somewhat distressed several months ago when I was told by a friend that when my name came up in a conversation, someone said, "Oh, yes, he's the obit writer for *GCN*." I consider myself a professional writer, capable of writing about anything that needs to be written. And when AIDS began hitting the gay community harder and harder, it seemed obvious that obituaries—of both "known" and "unknown" gay people—needed to be written. But in recent months I have to admit my sense of professionalism has been sorely strained by feelings of depression and inadequacy. Depression because there are so many obits that need to be written; inadequacy because the plain writing of obits was beginning to seem not enough. The litany of names, birth dates, death dates, diseases, lovers left, families left, what they did in their lives, what they did not do, and perhaps most of all, what any of this meant, was becoming unbearable because of its repetition.

After a while, writing became sentiment without feeling—an overload of funeral data that repeated death, death, death, but that did not help me, and possibly the readers, to *do* anything with the facts and what they signified.

In the past three years, I have become fairly obsessed with reading obits. I turn to them first when I open a paper. At the beginning of the epidemic, AIDS itself was hardly ever mentioned in obits, but you could usually assume the cause of death by the age or occupation and the ambiguous statements that the person died after a "long illness," or a "short illness." Recently, more and more obits admit to AIDS: It is a small comfort of progress. On a good day, there may not be any. The worst are when you actually know someone who has died, especially when you have had little or no warning. This happened to me with Gerald Chapman.

Clipping obits from *The New York Times* or the Boston *Globe* has become almost rote. They sit on my desk, or on the living room couch, as though in some nether world—no longer part of a newspaper but not yet anything else. Most of the time, I mean to use them to write obituaries for *GCN;* sometimes they just remain there, to be filed away or just serve as a reminder (as if one was needed) that AIDS is a daily part of life.

Many times, writing obits is not only depressing but distressing as well. It used to be reflexive, almost a writing exercise. Now it is impossible not to take it more personally, to see larger patterns, to feel threatened and insecure.

I also feel a sense of loss, which, ironically enough, is stronger if the lives I am reading about are not known to me. In mourning the loss of a friend, one is left with the resonance of that friendship. Noting the death of a faceless gay man with only a name and a few facts about his life on newsprint leaves me with a greater sense of loss since there is nothing to connect the obituary to the rest of my life.

These five obits—lives—are of gay men who were prominent in the arts: actors, dancers, directors, producers, artists, and photographers. I was only actually friends with one of them, but looking at them all together, typing out the list of names and the dates (one of them born the year before I was, one just a year later) is a painful experience. The pain comes not so much from the memento mori factor—although that is present in every-thing gay men do these days—but from realizing the sense of loss, devastating loss, which accompanies both the listing and the noting of all of these passings. The loss affects both the gay male community and gay male art in the world today.

The Stonewall Riots, which heralded the advent of gay libera-tion, came at a time when many postwar babies were beginning to realize their visions. It was also a time when U.S. culture was breaking out of the narrow social strictures of the 1950s. The arts especially were blooming: Off-Broadway, experimental theater, happenings, and new forms of dance and art exemplified this growth. There was an excitement and an encouragement from both the critics and the public for adventurous exploration in self-expression and artistic creativity. Gay male artists were at the forefront of many of these movements. Off-Broadway and Off-Off-Broadway would never have developed without the efforts and visions of gay men. The same is true of dance and many of the plastic arts, as well as music and performance work.

Peter Hujar started his career as a fashion photographer and later turned to fine-arts pictures and portraits. Some of his ear-liest pictures were of gay people in the arts: Charles Ludlam, Divine, William Burroughs. *Christopher Street* printed many of the photos, which were later collected, along with the artist's other photos of Mexican catacombs, in a volume entitled *Portraits in Life and Death*. Susan Sontag wrote the introduction to the book and praised the photographer's vision and sen-sitivity to both his subjects and his art. Hujar photos paved the way for the public acceptance of such gay artists as Robert Mapplethorpe and Arthur Tress.

Choo San Goh was the artistic director of the prestigious Washington Ballet when he died. His first work was presented by the Dutch National Ballet, for which he danced in 1973. He created dances for ballet and modern dance companies in Australia, Hong Kong, Sweden, Chile, and Israel. He also produced works for the Dance Theater of Harlem, the Alvin Ailey American Dance Theater, and the Boston Ballet. Goh and several other choreographers changed the aesthetic of ballet in the early Eighties. By combining idioms of modern dance and the structures of classical ballet, he created a new look that was both streamlined and accessible to a wide audience. Born in Singapore, Goh was influenced by the traditions of Asian dance as well, some of which he combined in a modernized form with traditional concepts of Western ballet.

Gerald Chapman got his start directing the Gay Sweatshop Theatre in London (a fact not mentioned in his *New York Times* obit). He also worked in London's Royal Court Theatre as the director of the Young Writer's Festival. He was then invited to America by Stephen Sondheim to start a similar project in New York. In 1983, Chapman and the Young Playwright's Festival of New York both won a Drama Critics Circle Award. In 1984–1985, he worked at the American Repertory Theater in Cambridge, developing scripts and directing the Monday-night series at the Hasty Pudding. Chapman always said his time at the Gay Sweatshop taught him how to work with actors in a more sensitive manner. The exhilaration of working with gay actors and breaking down social taboos in dealing with gay content was also creatively liberating for Chapman.

Barry Laine was one of the senior editors of *Stagebill* magazine and a contributing editor to *Dance Magazine*. But he will be remembered most for helping establish The Glines, New York's first gay theater and arts center. Along with John Glines, Laine helped produce a wealth of plays and readings by gay writers— the most famous of which were Harvey Firestein's *Torch Song Trilogy* and William Hoffman's *As Is*. Gay theater, as we know it today, is taken by many audiences as a given. Many do not realize that in the early Seventies it was Laine's and others'

work—the fundraising, the casting calls, the backstage drudg-
ery, and the endless promotional work necessary to get any press
attention whatsoever—that made gay theater a reality today.

Jerry Carlson was the principal conductor of the Los Angeles
Gay Men's Chorus between 1981 and 1987. He had lived in Los
Angeles since 1980, when he moved from Chicago, where he was
a charter member of the Chicago Gay Pride Band and cofounder
of the Windy City Chorus. He was also the cofounder of the Gay-
Lesbian Association of Choruses. While many other art forms are
limited in their audience appeal, the rise in the number of gay and
lesbian choruses throughout the country has posited an important move to musical popularism: a community-centered cultural
expression which is immediately inspiring and uplifting. It
would be impossible to separate Jerry Carlson, his music, and his
political work from the reality of an ever-increasing sense of gay
community and gay expression today.

Looking over these names and these achievements, it is impossible for me not to think of the many people who have died
of AIDS we have not read about, not heard about, and who are
mourned only by their friends. For each of these artists, there
are many more—stagehands, scene painters, singers, dancers,
actors, tech workers, designers, and gofers—we have lost.
These are the hidden deaths, but in a real sense they matter
even more. For although these five men had the good luck to
make names for themselves, it was the hard work of these
countless others which allowed them to reach the top. Every
now and then, there will be a piece in *Time, Newsweek, New
York Magazine*, or *Harper's* about the effect of AIDS on the artistic community. All of the usual names are called up—some of
these men will now be among them—but for the most part,
these articles miss the point. They are predicated on viewing
the death of an important artist from AIDS as a tragedy for the
arts world. That may be true. The more sobering fact is that it
is not just the death of a Peter Hujar or a Gerald Chapman
which affects their artistic communities—it is the death of any-

one working in those communities. The cost in talent, expertise, energy, and morale is incalculable. We do not know what that cost is now—living in the middle of the battlefield—and may not know for many years to come.

Writing this makes me realize how frightened I am—not so much of AIDS and death and all of the attending anxieties, but frightened of what is going to become of gay artists and gay culture in the next decade. We are not only losing some of our best talents—talents which came of age and matured during a very special period of artistic history—but we are also forced to create under a new and emotionally straining social and political environment inseparable from the epidemic.

I don't think for one minute that gay culture and gay sensibility are going to die out because of AIDS—we are too adaptable and innovative ever to allow that to happen. But I am worried that because of social, medical, and emotional forces beyond our control we will be forced to create in self-defense, in reaction *to* the epidemic and the conservative political backlash it has unleashed, rather than finding inspiration from our inner selves. I am also worried that the foothold gay men and lesbians have made in the arts—both in the mainstream popular culture and specially gay environments—will be lost. It will either be given up because we are too busy surviving and mourning, or taken away because of homophobia and public censure.

But despite the terrors of writing and reading obits, there is also the satisfaction, however incomplete, that something is being done. Someone's life has been noted. Some attention is being paid. Someone else may read and understand a little more of how large, how inclusive and diverse the gay world is. Most importantly, though, it is the very act of doing something, anything, in the face of AIDS that matters.

And in taking such action—as well in remembering and mourning, which are part of each obituary—the pieces ease both the terror and the pity, and they become politically inseparable from the personal.

All Too Familiar

MAREA MURRAY

I have passed the twenty people mark; more than twenty friends and acquaintances I've known are now dead from AIDS. Struggling for words to express the mix of feelings and numbness, I hear myself tell people, "Something's broken inside." I don't know what it means yet.

A social worker with intravenous-drug-using families, I go from a meeting to discuss one of my clients—a child with ARC—to another hospital to visit a friend diagnosed two weeks ago. Bill, a man in my pod of buddies at the AIDS Action Committee here in Boston, was admitted with *Pneumocystis* pneumonia and meningitis. Flowers in hand, I arrive to see him again, wondering how I'll find him, worried about the degree of pain I'd heard over the phone line.

Last week, my friend Katie went with me to see him. The sign on the door indicated that we should wear masks and gowns. We walked in and asked whether we should put them on. He said whatever would make us comfortable, so we sat down *sans*. He seemed okay, maybe in a bit of shock, talking a lot. The Walk for Life was the next day and he'd been given the walkie-talkie he would have carried as a marshal, so he could tune in. While we were there, they left his lunch tray outside the room. We were outraged. *This is nineteen fucking eighty-eight.*

Today, I get off the elevator. I had written about a man I called "Leo" in "Battles Joined: Odyssey of a Lesbian AIDS Activist," a series published in *Gay Community News*.* He stands at the end of the hall. Bill is dead, he says. He died at 10 A.M. They think it was a blood clot.

I hear myself saying Oh my God over and over. The tears rise and then return to their ducts. I am amazed at my thoughts: "Good, it was quick; he didn't suffer too long. . . ." I wonder how his parents will be about this terrible blow; he was their only child, a teddy bear sort of man. And I walk out through the lobby of this all-too-familiar hospital, into the day and the busy streets. It's strange to walk out with flowers. . . .

He is the third friend to die this month. Jane, my client with AIDS, is in the hospital with unexplained fevers. Jane's child, who I've been trying to get into day care for months, is being cared for by her adolescent sister, who is sullen and lost in the shuffle. I must tell Jane (I've changed the names of the people with whom I work, to protect their confidentiality) that I am leaving my job, but decide this is not a good time for me; maybe I'm in shock or, worse yet, "getting used to it."

So I walk to my car with the lavender and gold sticker FIGHT AIDS NOT PEOPLE WITH AIDS, wondering for the umpteenth time if and when I'll find it vandalized because of the sticker. I get in and tell myself to let the tears fall. I smell the flowers and close my eyes.

Seated, motionless, I notice that the black interior holds the sun. I am happy it is summer finally and the light beats down on me. I flash to Jane asking me the other day, point blank, if I "go with girls"—after beating around the bush, asking if I work on Saturday. Maybe I could give her a ride home from the hospital if they let her out. What do I do on weekends anyway? Do I have a boyfriend? I smile and start the car. I will remember her that way, too.

Gay Community News, Vol. 15, Nos. 29–33.

Her grin at my yes answer is triumphant. She reminds me of Rita, with whom I was buddies years ago. "I knew it," Jane says gleefully. Her best friend "in the whole world" is "like that." She's in prison and Jane has missed her. "This'll bring us closer," she says to me. I haven't the heart to tell her I'm leaving this work, this so-direct service with people with AIDS (PWAs) and IV users. Next time. I will enjoy Jane's laughter and stories instead.

All in a week. Years into this epidemic—four and a half for me—and it feels like a lifetime.

My thoughts drift back to my first meeting with her, "my PWA client." It was a cold afternoon a couple of months ago. I'd been to see Michael, another friend with AIDS from AIDS Action days. He was having trouble breathing, probably going in again, and I'd wanted to see him for some time, putting it off because I knew . . . I knew the closer I got to him, the harder the pain would be to bear, watching him go. We talked, hugged, and were silent together. He showed me photos of his lover, Abel, who'd died years ago with AIDS. Then he showed me a photo of his current girlfriend. His buddy, a woman, arrived as I bid him farewell. I worried about squeezing him too tightly, given his frail condition.

Back to work, I went to do an intake on a woman, an IV-drug user suspected of having AIDS, like most of our clients requesting help with day care. Her doctor called while I was there. It was confirmed; Jane had AIDS.

She was sobbing. Her children were asleep in the other room, and the television was on. This is a goddamn intake I screamed inside, furious that she'd gotten the word over the phone. I held her, tried to comfort her, hold the horror away. Bill got his news over the phone, too. All too familiar . . .

"This means I'm going to die, doesn't it?"

She told her teenage daughter, who broke down. I asked myself what I was doing there—a white social worker, witnessing the grief of a black family I had never met before. I told myself, yes, and it's happening all over. I shrugged when a roommate asked how my day had been and I said "surreal" because that's what it felt like.

In June, Michael and Bill are both dead. One struggled for years, the other for weeks. My clients continue to struggle—Jane and her children, the women who hope they and their children will not become ill, who battle the dangers of the needle and everything else. The stories from Stockholm, the site of the 1988 international AIDS conference, fuel my dreams of fire; I dream of bodies stacked like those of the Holocaust and I recognize these faces. I have not slept through the night in weeks.

I will leave this work at the end of the month. The NAMES Project's Quilt is visiting Boston. Tears flood me as I enter the building. The "no more names" slogan seems curious to me. There will be names for years to come. I marvel at the beauty of my friend Bob's panel until I see Abel and Michael's below it. Then I sob in my friend's arms. Bill's wake was last night in a Boston suburb; a few of us went so there'd be a gay presence. But his parents blame the doctors for missing the blood clot. AIDS is not mentioned. His work as a buddy is not mentioned. It is all too familiar.

Many men I know have lost close friends and lovers, numbering in the double digits. I feel estranged and alone in the women's community and I joke that I am of a different species, isolated even among many lesbian friends and roommates. I'm able to ask for hugs when I need them, but that is not enough. I am drowning in grief when I let myself feel it, wondering what price is being exacted from my health and sanity, and those of my friends and other AIDS workers/activists.

Multiple deaths are not new to me. Some of this grief probably stems from my experiences as a survivor. I witnessed my father's death, his experimental treatments, and the ordeals of my relatives who have died with cancer.

And now it's my friends, my buddies, and my clients. People ask me how I do it. I don't know. I know I must rest. So I stop going to meetings. I write about other things; I go dancing; I take long baths; I go to movies; I love my friends. And I wonder.

I wonder who will be next. I wonder how many of my clients will become ill. A part of me doesn't want to know. A part of me does, wants to keep in touch, keep fighting. I analyze it to death.

I wonder if I'm burned out, if I will break down at my next Women and AIDS presentation. But something tells me I've gone beyond that—"over the top." Over twenty seems to be a marker. I gave my first eulogy at twenty-five. I read the obituaries as regularly as I do the comics. That's how I found out about Michael. Crying, I ask no one in particular when this will end. Not in my lifetime. I am twenty-eight.

It's not supposed to be like this. But it is. Relentless. And I must nurture myself to keep going—to hospital rooms, funeral homes, memorial services, and the rest. I know I have never valued life as much as I do with each passing day. Life is far too short and precious to waste or burn. Perhaps I'll feel more sane tomorrow. It's another day, after all.

Memorial Day, 1988

ROBERT DAWIDOFF

1.

Michael Denneny was saying that he was being interviewed frequently these days concerning the new writing about AIDS. One thing people kept asking that angered him and made him think for a reply was about the aesthetic worth of this new literature. *Was it really good, would it last, what were its merits, artistically speaking?* And he, an intellectual, gay, an editor, was distressed about an answer. We were talking it over. One thing we came to was just to question the importance of form in registering agony; is there a beautiful way to scream in pain? Of course there is in opera, and the question always comes back to the old one about art and life. How much verismo can we stand in life?

The quips come easy:

INTERVIEWER: . . . but, Mr. Denneny, will this literature about AIDS last?

*   *   *

MR. DENNENY: The way things are going, it is bound to outlast its audience. . . .

But once you begin to think about it, a hard thought dawns. AIDS has indeed changed the relation of art to life and has created and recreated forms and genres that obviate our assumptions about *culture,* which is what monitors our agreements about what art has to do with life and life with art. AIDS threatens all the institutions and assumptions about art and life that amount to the institutions of culture. It throws a wrench into the machinery of cultural reflection.

2.

AIDS is a matter of life and death. The way literature has to do with life and death is complicated, but forms develop to cover most eventualities. Memorial and elegy and raging against the dying of the light, the beating of breasts and the tenderest emotions of loss relate us to the eventual, the unavoidable, the natural, the inexplicable. They accustom us to our feelings and ennoble our responses. They comfort us and keep us company. They soothe and guide our participation in the human condition. But AIDS has forced these conventions into unseasonal flower. One poem to a dead youth or a child mourned by a parent focuses the reversal of the natural order of things. AIDS has made a rule of this exception and made what tradition regarded as unspeakably sad or terrible into a daily experience.

The horror of war is the collective loss and it is soothed by patriotism or bitterness, but it has the backing of the collectivity, which is reasserted through memorial. A generation "lost" becomes a generation mourned, remembered by surviving comrades and descendants, who will take the country over in their turn. If we wait for AIDS to be over, who will be left to mourn? It is killing our collectivity.

AIDS speeds up remembrance. People in their youth are having to remember their youth, as death and the ravages of the disease destroy their memories, the memories of their foreshortened lives. What are the aesthetics of this need to remember in order to live a little longer and to die a little better? What are the forms of the terrible, plaguing, releasing, enlivening, dying anger, the rage against more than the dying of the light?

The writing about AIDS reports from the thing itself. It unsettles all the assumptions culture codifies about how art is supposed to work and how long it is supposed to take for it to work and who decides whether what is working is really art.

3.

AIDS has vitalized writing. Volunteerism has become a principle of reading and writing about medicine and science, as the institutions of scientific truth and medicine in the society have failed people with or at risk for AIDS. Writing spreads the words about AIDS and encourages the healing, educating, caring, researching, nursing, supporting, organizing jobs among the population that the institutionalized systems of science and government and culture have not. It forces the present. Ringing out danger, ringing out a warning.

*   *   *

Every aspect of life has had to be written about. AIDS has made specific truth about our lives and deaths the basic stake of writing. And we have learned that it cannot be left up to doctors and scientists and newspapers and preachers and politicians. If writing about AIDS is not true, the interested reader is going to know it, to find it out. The relative truth of a piece of writing, a kind of writing, has become more of an issue. The way in which we read has changed. Letting fashion and other people decide what is true and useful and should be written and published has turned out to be dangerous and endangering. The intensity with which we have come to read about health, diet, sex, politics, and spirit has affected us as readers of literature. We need it more, and we demand more from it and we know it when we read it, know it for ourselves.

And who *we* are is changing, too; we are more disparate and more variously affected and brought together by AIDS. *We* are who decides to be affected by AIDS. And literature has had to do with making us so.

AIDS has created political writing in which reflection has had to inform and energize action and action right now. It has compressed observation, journalism, political thinking, propaganda, and strategy into a literature of political immediacy that can make common realities clear and suggest courses of action to keep the community going through hell on earth. Think of what writing has accomplished in the last several years in terms of national organizations, dissemination of survival information, literature of the spirit, history, "how to" and "how not to" books on all levels—writing about our very lives to save them.

* * *

Anne Frank's diary had its own special beauty, but it was written without her really knowing what would happen, and we read it knowing there is nothing we can do about it. AIDS writing is about something we know is happening and about which we must, in fact, do something. It is about all the things we can do and feel. It is a literature of discovery. It is engaged and activist writing, and its truth and beauties will not wait on academics or posterity for judgment. Posterity is just around the corner.

The reader and writer community of AIDS has rediscovered the social roots of any kind of writing, the roots in human survival, expression, ritual, and need. We need to have these things written. The information, the truth, the anger, the philosophy, the history, the fiction, the poetry, the spirituality do a job now. Their place in history will be judged by their success in helping to keep the community that the writing serves alive, safer, together, comforted in sickness and in loss, defended against persecution.

4.

What AIDS has done is to reacquaint a community with the expressive function in human life. No community has had to do so many artistic things, for their original purposes, so quickly and for such pressing reasons. AIDS writing cannot only be gay literature—or gay and lesbian literature—although the gay community is at the heart of AIDS and is one model for what AIDS means. The two are not synonymous. Still, AIDS is a fact of gay history, and the most intense communal loss has been the gay loss.

*　　*　　*

The Nazis killed many people, but the symbolic focus of the Holocaust is its systematic slaughter of the Jews. *Never again.* But holocausts do not necessarily happen again to the same people in the same way. The studies of the Holocaust demonstrate the necessity of being aware of something while it is going on, overcoming denial, of recognizing that the pariah community must fight back and refuse to deceive itself, must refuse to be intimidated and victimized. This plague feels political, it occasions wider persecutions, and we can only learn from the history that we know.

Genocide does not ever happen in the same way to the same people, but it always means the wiping out of a despised people through active malevolence or the manipulation of the accidental, plus the denial of its targeted community, and the indifference of the world and its acquiescence in the horror. AIDS has forced gay people to consider the unthinkable. It is not to say this *is* a holocaust, to say that AIDS has made us have to consider the possibility along with everything else and to extend our thinking and writing to this ghastly eventuality as well.

And we need the stories, the feelings, the situations, the characters, the adventure, the humor, the romance, the memories, and the affirmation of the recent sexual and communal and emotional past that novels and poets can give us. We need the stories the AIDS Memorial Quilt collected. We need the voices of PWAs, the stories of the tending and the tended. We need our formidable imaginations and the resources of our style, our aesthetic sense, our sexual memories, as much as we need our other resources. We need what makes life good. We need to rescue our loves from all this trouble.

What Michael will have to say next time in answer to that frustrating question is that the literature on AIDS has recovered the purpose of art. It is the intelligent, various, activated response of a people's expressive immune system to an epidemic threat. Its power is primary, its timetable immediate—and its purpose is action, the action of healing, curing, organizing, comforting, understanding, surviving, dying, remembering, loving—every conceivable human action is its business.

If aesthetics amounts to something different from this, if aesthetics requires the recapitulation at a distance of present agony, if aesthetics means the contemplation in form, from a distance, then we must be brave and risk aesthetic failure. But we who read the literature of AIDS do not believe so and who publishes it does not think so. If we all do our part, there may even be time to talk about the aesthetics after a while. With any luck.

NOTES ON
THE CONTRIBUTORS

STEVE BEERY is a freelance journalist and essayist. He has written extensively for *The Advocate*, and his work has appeared in *Interview, Vanity Fair, The Pink Paper* (London), and the San Francisco *Chronicle*. He is the recipient of a 1981 Cable Car Award, and is among those profiled in Frances FitzGerald's *Cities on a Hill*. He lives in San Francisco.

MICHAEL BRONSKI is a writer whose film, theater, and literary criticism, as well as articles on sexuality, have appeared in the Boston *Globe, Fag Rag, Z Magazine, The Advocate, Gay Community News*, and *The Boston Phoenix*. He is the author of *Culture Clash: The Making of a Gay Sensibility* and has contributed pieces to many anthologies. He has been a gay activist for twenty years.

STEPHEN M. CHAPOT was born November 21, 1951. He was raised in Millbrae, California, and San Francisco. He attended San Francisco State University and the University of California's medical illustrating program in the 1970s. He was diagnosed with AIDS while working as an illustrator in Los Angeles. "Liz Taylor, Live!" was the first in a series of published writings describing his experiences. His writing, along with a number of public speeches and a great body of drawings and graphics, has become his legacy.

ROBERT DAWIDOFF chairs the history department at the Claremont Graduate School, where he also codirects American Studies. Among his publications are *The Education of John Randolph* and the forthcoming *The Genteel Tradition and the Sacred Rage.* His writings have appeared in *The Advocate, The London Review of Books,* Los Angeles *Times,* and many other popular periodicals and scholarly journals.

ROBERT GLÜCK's most recent books are *Reader,* poems and short prose, and *Jack the Modernist,* a novel. He is an activist and the director of the Poetry Center at San Francisco State University.

E. J. GRAFF is a writer and editor who lives in the Boston area. Her articles, essays, poems, and reviews have been published in *Bay Windows, Sojourner, The Women's Review of Books, The American Voice, The Boston Phoenix,* and elsewhere. She won a 1988 Massachusetts Artists Foundation Award in Poetry and has been a fellow at both Yaddo and the MacDowell Colony.

STEPHEN GRECO is Deputy Arts editor for *7 Days* and for three years was New York editor of *The Advocate.* He has written often on gay life.

ANDREW HOLLERAN is the author of the novels *Dancer from the Dance* and *Nights in Aruba,* and a book of essays on AIDS, *Ground Zero.*

ARNIE KANTROWITZ is an associate professor of English at the College of Staten Island, City University of New York. His essays have appeared in *The Advocate, The Village Voice,* London's *Gay News, The New York Times,* and other publications. His poetry has appeared in *Trace, Descant, The Mouth of the Dragon,* and other literary magazines. He is the author of an autobiography, *Under the Rainbow: Growing Up Gay,* and he has recently completed a novel about a modern disciple of Walt Whitman.

MAREA MURRAY, L.I.C.S.W., is a therapist in Boston, Massachusetts. An AIDS activist and caregiver since January of 1984, she has published a five-part series, "Battles Joined: Odyssey of a Lesbian AIDS Activist," in *Gay Community News* and an essay, "Women Included," in Cleis Press's anthology *AIDS: The Women,* as well as several articles on safer sex for lesbian and bisexual women.

JOHN PRESTON is the author of numerous books, including *Franny, the Queen of Provincetown* and the Alex Kane adventure novels. The former editor of *The Advocate,* he has written extensively about AIDS and about sexuality during the epidemic (he coauthored *Safe Sex: The Ultimate Erotic Guide* with Glenn Swann). He lives in Portland, Maine, and is currently working on a gay resource guide and a commentary on the sex industry.

CRAIG ROWLAND is a New York journalist whose articles about AIDS, the arts, and other subjects appear in *The Advocate* and other publications.

LAURENCE TATE lives in San Francisco and volunteers with several AIDS organizations. Over the years, he has written articles for *Arrival, Body Politic,* and other publications. He continues to write about AIDS and is working on a book about his experiences in the sixties.

ALLAN TROXLER teaches English country dance, free of the traditional men's and women's roles, and works as a graphic artist and yardsman.

SCOTT TUCKER is a writer and activist whose work has appeared in *Christopher Street*, *The New York Native*, *Gay Community News*, *The Advocate*, *Body Politic*, and other publications. He is currently working on a book combining politics and autobiography.

EDMUND WHITE is a contributing editor to *Artforum*. He has written several novels, including *A Boy's Own Story* and *The Beautiful Room Is Empty*. He is now writing a biography of Jean Genet.